Professor Gerard

Polycystic Ovary Syndrome

Your Medical Handbook

Published by Munday Books 2016

First published in Great Britain in 2016 by Munday Books

ISBN 978-0-9563297-1-4

Cover Design by Tim Foster

Typeset by Hope Services (Abingdon) Ltd

Printed and bound in Great Britain by
CPI Anthony Rowe

about the author

Professor Gerard Conway is a Reproductive Endocrinologist at University College London Hospitals with an academic base in the Institute for Women's Health, University College London. His association with PCOS dates back to 1987 when he first started clinics 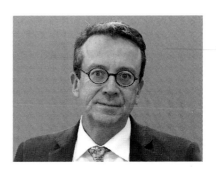 at the Middlesex Hospital under one of the pioneers of reproductive endocrinology – Professor Howard Jacobs. As a research fellow he subsequently performed studies on the importance of insulin resistance and inheritance patterns in PCOS. This work formed the basis of a doctorate thesis at the University of London.

Over the ensuing years, Professor Conway has met many hundreds of women with PCOS covering all aspects of treatment relating to both androgens and fertility. It is this experience that is now laid down in the words contained in this book.

Clinical research in reproductive endocrinology undertaken by Professor Conway has been the presented around the world at meetings of learned societies. His expertise is documented in over 200 publications including, as co-editor, an academic book on PCOS.

about the artist

Myrto Williams is a freelance illustrator and specialises in working with people, particularly children, to develop and facilitate workshops and events that explore connections between art, science and society. She has worked alongside institutions such as the British Museum and Imperial College London.

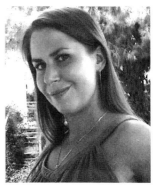

Myrto graduated from Camberwell College of Arts in 2010 with a BA in Illustration. In all of her creative work and professional experience she explores creativity as a tool for self-expression and a means to motivate both oneself and others.

She is currently undertaking a MA in Child and Adolescent Psychotherapy while also working at a Special Needs Secondary School. In this way she continues to explore the need for visual expression as a means to understand and aid emotional and physical well-being.

www.myrto-williams.com

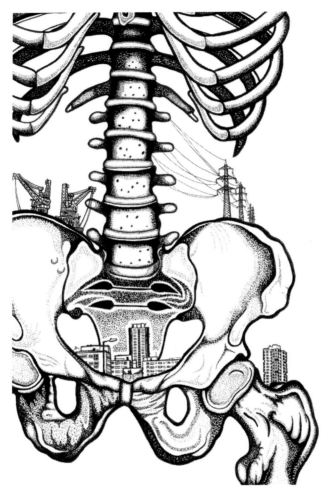

Support System

a favourite from the gallery of Myrto Williams

contents

illustrations

graphs

foreword

what is in a book about PCOS?

I remember when, as a junior doctor, I suggested to a senior colleague that I envisaged a career investigating the cause and consequences of PCOS. I was strongly advised against such a plan on the basis that it was a poorly defined condition and that it would be ultimately frustrating to work in an area with layers of uncertainty; not least because no one could define exactly what the syndrome was! Despite having great respect for this professor, I embarked on research into PCOS starting with the interplay between the hormone insulin and the ovary. My first research project in PCOS was in the 1980s. It involved testing hormone profiles in over 100 women with PCOS together with their parents. This research showed how much we each inherit traits such as weight and insulin levels from our parents.

Alongside the laboratory research, my outpatient clinics became a constant source of learning. Over the next 20 years I met many women with PCOS and constantly adjusted thoughts on treatment and lifestyle in the light of experience and feedback from patients. In this book I have tried to put into some order the discussions that I have had with my patients together with those that I have had with researchers and colleagues in the field.

My background is in conventional medicine which is the basis of most of the information in this book. I hope that I have been able to achieve my goal of providing detailed medical information that is easily accessible to someone without a degree in biology! At times it has been hard to decide what to include and what to leave out. I have opted to keep the level quite high on the basis that anyone with a lifelong condition benefits from maximum information. In fact, it might be thought that this book was intended for doctors. While medical practitioners may well find the book useful, my main aim was to provide a reference of medical information for women with PCOS so that they had access to the same knowledge base as doctors.

The idea of a handbook is that this might be something that you can dip in and out of depending on circumstance. Because the label PCOS covers such a wide spectrum, not everything in this book will apply to you. On the other hand, as time passes problems relating to PCOS can change so other sections may become relevant later on. Even though there is a great deal of information available on the Internet and in various self-help books, many of my patients have said how difficult it is to work out where they fit into the wider picture. I hope that somewhere in this book the readers may gain a perspective relevant to their own experience of PCOS.

Words only get you so far. I noticed that many books on PCOS lacked the diagrams that I find helpful when describing how the body works (and misbehaves!). I have been greatly assisted by Myrto Williams who has patiently provided content for illustrations. Women who have attended my clinics may well recognize some of these diagrams that I use in clinic in order to understand the processes involved and how different treatments work.

The information in this volume is based on my personal opinion and other doctors will differ in their assessment of different treatments. For instance, those with a background in gynaecology tend to focus only on fertility, whereas those with a background in general practice or endocrinology think about PCOS in terms of the effect of testosterone on the skin and management of irregular periods. I have been fortunate enough to be a physician working in a department of women's health and I hope therefore to have been able to cover both spheres of influence.

I am conscious that one difficulty with putting all of this information down in printed form is that it may quickly go out of date. New research is adding to our knowledge base all of the time. Similarly, regulations come and go regarding treatments that may be available at any one time – they also vary depending on where you live. It may be that some treatments mentioned in this book are not readily available to you. I realize that this can open up a frustration of a hope that cannot be fulfilled – for this I apologize.

In summary, I hope that this book fills a gap in the information that is not widely available from other sources. I would be interested to hear from any reader who has a comment.

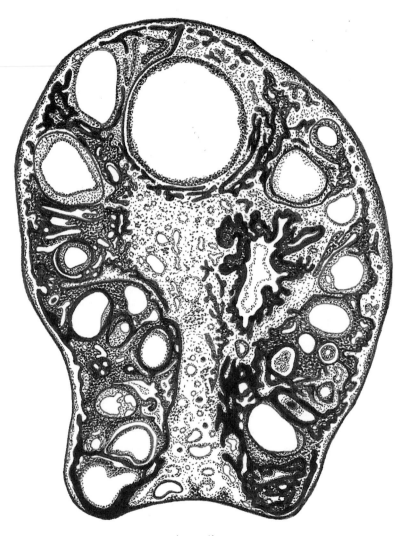

a polycystic ovary

This is a line drawing of a section through the ovary interpreted from a histological specimen. On the outside there is a series of follicles of different sizes. The follicle largest at the top is approaching the size of a dominant follicle ready for ovulation. Below and to the left of this is a collapsing corpus luteum left over from a previous cycle. The centre of the ovary is called the medulla where the nerves and blood vessels supply the ovary.

chapter 1
introduction and a bit of history

what is PCOS?

Polycystic ovary syndrome is the most common cause of irregular periods and unwanted hair growth in women. It affects about 1 in 10 of all women. PCOS can show itself any time after puberty when the ovaries become most active.

The word *polycystic* is made up of the Greek word *poly* meaning many and the medical term *cysts* which describes small sacs filled with fluid. Follicles are the little cyst-like areas in the ovary where eggs develop. Follicles come and go within the ovary and on average there are about eight visible at any one time. In polycystic ovaries there are more than 12 follicles in each ovary. It would be more accurate to say 'polyfollicle' ovary instead of polycystic but we are stuck with a historic name.

In addition to having more follicles than average, the polycystic ovary also makes more than the average amount of the male hormone *testosterone* which is present in all women in small amounts. It is testosterone that causes most of the mischief in PCOS such as acne and unwanted hair growth. The symptoms of PCOS become worse with weight gain and therefore problems arise more commonly for women who are overweight. Throughout this book, the effects of being overweight will be a common theme.

A distinction is often made between polycystic ovaries which are seen on an ultrasound scan and polycystic ovary

<u>syndrome</u>. The ultrasound appearance of polycystic ovaries is common, occurring in about 20% of all women. Polycystic ovary <u>syndrome</u> is the combination of polycystic ovaries on ultrasound and a variety of symptoms such as unwanted hair growth, acne or infrequent periods. The syndrome occurs in about 10% of women or one half of those with PCO on ultrasound.

In this book we will explore all of the problems related to PCOS in detail as well as the treatments that are available.

an ultrasound image of a polycystic ovary

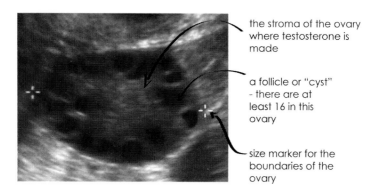

the stroma of the ovary where testosterone is made

a follicle or "cyst" - there are at least 16 in this ovary

size marker for the boundaries of the ovary

is PCOS a disease?

PCOS is not really a disease. Rather, it is a label that describes the way the ovaries are working. In some ways, PCOS can be considered a variation from normal – a label applied to a group of women whose ovaries are more active than average. The activity of the ovary is partly measured both by the number of follicles visible at any one time and partly by the amount of testosterone it makes. But most of all, it is measured by the symptoms related to it. When ovaries are being handed out, some women receive a 'quiet one' while others receive a more active polycystic one. The activity of the ovary is partly determined by the luck of the genes that are inherited and partly by lifestyle such as diet, exercise and bodyweight.

The activity level of the ovaries can be described in several ways. The most sensitive is by counting the number of follicles visible and measuring the overall size of the ovary using ultrasound. Also, the amount of testosterone in the blood can be measured but results from these tests are very variable and will be normal in many women with PCOS.

Another reason why PCOS is not like a disease is because it tends to gradually improve over life. For instance, the ovary is at its most active between the ages of 15 and 25 and from this time onwards the overall activity is reduced in all women. For women with PCOS, this means that some of the symptoms improve. In particular, periods that can be very irregular in the early 20s can become quite regular in women in their 40s. Unfortunately, other symptoms such as unwanted hair growth are less likely to get better over time.

the changing shape of PCOS in history

Many textbooks start a section on PCOS by making reference to bearded women in history as early examples of the condition. In particular, one woman with a beard who also had diabetes was on show in public exhibitions in the 1800s and the diabetes might have indicated a problem with the action of insulin that will be discussed later in this chapter.

The first time that the concept of PCOS was really pulled together was in 1935 in a paper by Stein and Leventhal who described a group of women with hirsutism, a complete lack of periods and very enlarged ovaries with multiple 'cysts'. This was the origin of the word cyst used for this syndrome. This was before the days of ultrasound scanning or even laparoscopes so the ovary appearance was discovered during an open operation. This was clearly a severe form of PCOS. The label *Stein and Leventhal Syndrome* continued to be used for the next 50 years. Key papers referred to in this section are summarised in Chapter 11.

a timeline showing how the concept of polycystic ovary syndrome has developed over time

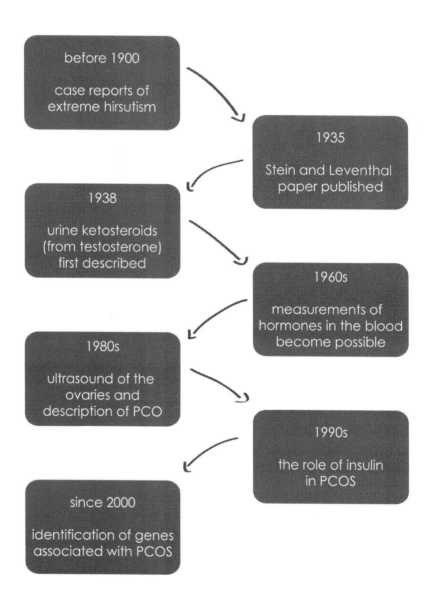

Through the 1960s and 70s measurements of various substances in the blood and in the urine became possible. Research on PCOS then focused on hormone testing which was fairly crude in the early years. First, testosterone and related compounds could be measured in the urine and were found to be raised in many women with PCOS. Another key hormone for PCOS is luteinising hormone which is made by the pituitary gland. This hormone could only usefully be measured in the blood requiring sensitive techniques that were developed in the late 1960s.

High-resolution ultrasound was a breakthrough technology that emerged in the 1980s which made it possible to obtain a good picture of the ovary for the first time. Before this, the structure of the ovary could only be closely examined directly by eye during an open operation or with a laparoscope. With ultrasound it was possible to count the number of follicles inside the ovary. It was very soon realised that approximately 20% of women fell into a group with more than the average number of follicles. Ultrasound helped to define the mild end of the spectrum of PCOS and turned what was previously considered to be an unusual condition into a very common one. In other words, the severe Stein and Leventhal syndrome was on one end of a very wide spectrum; at the very mild end of it are women with polycystic ovaries on ultrasound but who have none of the symptoms of PCOS and would otherwise consider themselves to be completely normal (they are!).

So the label 'PCOS' came to replace others terms. For example, the term 'idiopathic hirsutism' was previously applied to women with unwanted hair growth but normal blood tests, many of whom were found to have polycystic ovaries on ultrasound. Idiopathic hirsutism was effectively re-labeled as PCOS when ultrasound came along.

In the 1990s, medical researchers began to learn how PCOS and being overweight were linked. Much research effort was devoted to trying to work out whether it was the ovaries that caused weight gain or the other way round. The overall conclusion was that it was excess weight that made polycystic ovaries behave badly and that the hormone controlling this was insulin.

A proportion of women with PCOS, especially those with weight gain, were found to have a higher concentration of insulin in the circulation than average. The ovary is sensitive to an increase in insulin and responds by making more testosterone, therefore driving more symptoms to occur. The cause of raised insulin in the circulation was described as a condition called *insulin resistance*. Research on insulin also showed that women with PCOS were more likely to develop diabetes in pregnancy – known as *gestational diabetes* – and later in life, type 2 diabetes.

In the 2000s there was an explosion in genetic research in an effort to identify the genes that controlled the development of the ovary and why some ovaries were more active than others. It quickly became apparent that no single gene could account for the inheritance of PCOS. Instead, PCOS is thought to be caused by several genes. Some genes might affect how easily testosterone is made, others determine how sensitive the skin is in responding to testosterone and yet other genes will affect the action of insulin and the tendency to gain weight.

It is the luck of the draw when each person is made, whether PCO will develop. In some families the inheritance of PCOS is quite strong with several family members all experiencing symptoms. In others, it may be that only one woman inherits the trait. Because PCOS has such a wide spectrum of features, it requires many hundreds of women to take part in research projects in order to identify important genes. So far only a few genes have been found to be clearly related to PCOS.

how the ovary works

what is happening to hormones during the monthly cycle?

In order to understand some of the concepts discussed in this book it is useful to start with an overview of the reproductive system in women. The pituitary gland is the central controller of several hormone systems including the thyroid and adrenal glands and of course, the ovary. The pituitary gland makes two fertility hormones called gonadotrophins, one of which is luteinising hormone (LH) and the other is follicle-stimulating hormone (FSH). LH and FSH pass through the circulation to the ovaries where they drive the production of both hormones and eggs.

From a pool of eggs dormant within the ovary, FSH takes part in selecting a few that will begin to mature and from these a single dominant follicle grows, which is then selected for ovulation. Those follicles that do not make it the whole way to ovulation gradually die away. In this way, the ovary is constantly in a state of preparing new follicles for future cycles and allowing unused follicles to retire from the fertility process.

A follicle is made up of a central egg or oocyte surrounded by cells that make oestrogen and fluid that will gradually collect around the egg as the follicle grows – this is known as follicular fluid. This inner lining of cells is made up of granulosa cells. Around the granulosa cell is a different cell type called interstitial cells or theca cells. Theca cells are driven by LH to make testosterone. Testosterone is then taken up by the granulosa cell to be changed to oestrogen.

The first two weeks of the cycle is called the follicular phase as this is the time that the follicles grow and the amount of oestrogen and testosterone produced gradually rises to a peak at the time of ovulation. The dominant follicle is the one that is chosen for ovulation and it will grow from 5 mm to 20 mm as it matures – 2 mm per day! When the dominant

the pathway from pituitary to ovary

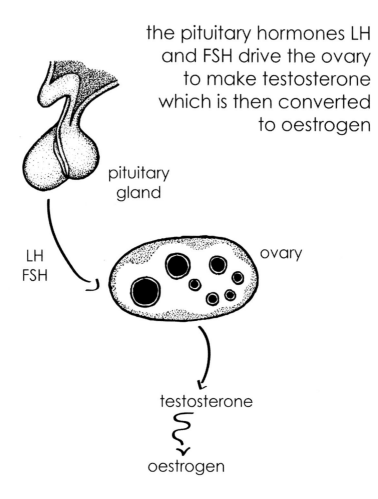

the pituitary hormones LH
and FSH drive the ovary
to make testosterone
which is then converted
to oestrogen

pituitary
gland

LH
FSH

ovary

testosterone

oestrogen

follicle is ready to burst for the egg to be released from the surface of the ovary, there is a surge of the hormone LH from the pituitary gland that triggers this ovulation.

If ovulation is successful then the follicle, from which the egg is released, collapses to form the corpus luteum. In this process the granulosa cells change in nature from making oestrogen to start making the hormone progesterone. This

a close-up of a follicle in the ovary

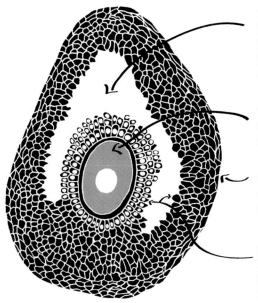

the middle of the follicle fills up with follicular fluid that forms the middle of a "cyst"

the egg or oocyte matures within the follicle

theca cells form an outer layer and make testosterone

granulosa cells form the inner layer of the follicle and convert testosterone to oestrogen

change defines the second half of the cycle called the luteal phase. Progesterone acts on the lining of the womb, called the endometrium to prepare it for implantation of an embryo if the egg has been fertilised. If no embryo appears then the progesterone level gradually declines and a period occurs. It is the hormone progesterone that causes many of the symptoms that we attribute to the premenstrual phase such as fluid retention, bloating and mood swings.

where does insulin fit in?

While the primary drive to the ovary is from the hormones LH and FSH, there is a secondary drive to the ovary by the hormone insulin. The main role of insulin is to control the

the surface of the ovary when cut through the middle

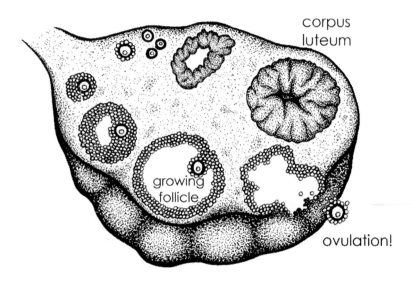

corpus luteum

growing follicle

ovulation!

level of the sugar glucose in the blood. It is a priority that the glucose level is held very precisely within a tight margin. The harder the body has to work to control glucose, the higher the level of insulin in the blood. For instance, in someone who is very overweight the body has to work hard to service the extra fat tissue and the level of insulin in the blood rises. By a curious feature of body design, the ovary is sensitive to the level of insulin, which stimulates the production of testosterone made by the ovary. The ovary, in turn, tends to misbehave more as weight goes up, while conversely the symptoms of PCOS improve as weight comes down.

Other factors can affect the level of insulin in the blood. Insulin levels go up if there is a high content of sugar and carbohydrates in the diet. Also, some families have an inherited tendency to run high insulin levels. The most important clue of this happening in a family is if there are several members with type 2 diabetes.

the monthly ovarian cycle

This diagram shows the maturing follicle at the top with ovulation on day 14 then the formation of a corpus luteum. A period starts on day 1 of the cycle and then the lining of womb thickens ready for the the embryo to implant. The hormone LH reaches a peak at ovulation and can be measured in urine as an ovulation test. Body temperature rises by about half a degree at ovulation.

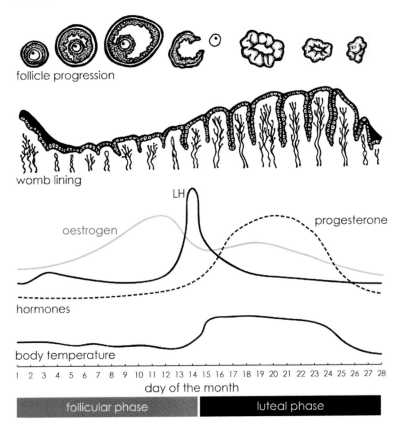

follicle progression

womb lining

LH

oestrogen

progesterone

hormones

body temperature

1 2 3 4 5 6 7 8 9 10 11 12 13 14 15 16 17 18 19 20 21 22 23 24 25 26 27 28
day of the month

follicular phase   luteal phase

insulin is a secondary drive to the ovary

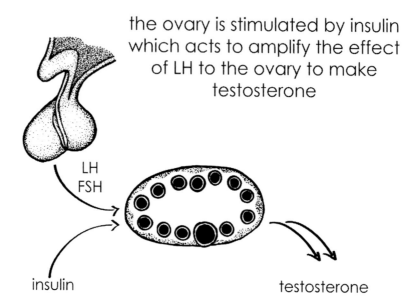

the ovary is stimulated by insulin which acts to amplify the effect of LH to the ovary to make testosterone

LH
FSH

insulin   testosterone

what happens to the eggs as I grow older?

The ovary is a unique organ in that it is programmed to survive for only about 50 years. For women trying to conceive, it is important to understand the ageing process of the ovary. The summary that follows applies to all women with or without PCOS. The ageing process for the ovary and the age of the menopause is about the same for women with PCOS and those without. In chapter 8 we go into the process of the menopause relating to women with PCOS in more detail.

A woman is born with all of the eggs that she will ever have in life. From birth onwards, no new eggs are ever made.

At birth, there are approximately one million eggs in each ovary. By some mysterious mechanism these eggs are constantly being tested for their quality. If there is any doubt as to whether the egg will be healthy for later use – perhaps in 30 years time, then it is dispatched for destruction. This process called programmed cell death occurs throughout life until the ovary finally runs out of eggs at approximately the age of 50 which is the average age for menopause. Between 25 and 100 eggs are destroyed in this way every day! If a woman were to ovulate every month between the age of 15 and 50 then fewer than 500 eggs would ever be released. In other words 4999 out of every 5000 eggs are destined for destruction! Or, to put it another way, only 0.05% of eggs are used for ovulation.

the number of eggs in the ovary over a lifetime

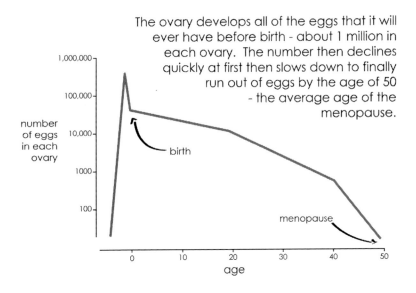

When a woman is in her late 30s the declining number of eggs can become critical. This can be the reason for age-related infertility. This is also the reason why women should try to start their families before the age of 35 and complete their family by the age of 38. The older the egg, the higher the risk of miscarriage and the less likely it is that the egg will fertilise. In addition, it can be difficult to make the ovary ovulate if only a small number of eggs remain. This age-related infertility is referred to as *low ovarian reserve*.

the chances of conceiving with advancing age

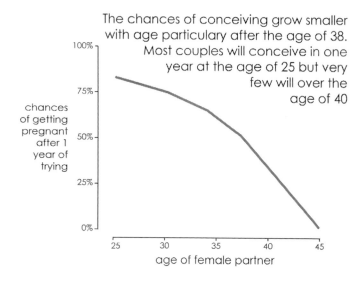

The chances of conceiving grow smaller with age particulary after the age of 38. Most couples will conceive in one year at the age of 25 but very few will over the age of 40

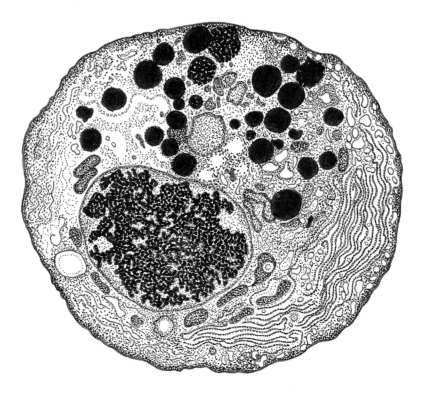

insulin-secreting beta cell of the pancreas

This is a schematic of the cell in the pancreas that makes insulin.
The darkest areas are secretory granules that store insulin ready for
release. When the cell receives the correct signal, these granules
move to the surface of the cell and burst open so that insulin is
released into the bloodstream. The nucleus is on the lower left
portion of the cell – this contains the genetic material that controls
the protein production. On the right-hand side is an organelle called
the Golgi apparatus where insulin is made before being packaged
into the granules. It is estimated that there are one million of these
cells in the pancreas.

chapter 2
making the diagnosis

how is PCOS defined by doctors?

Most of the time, the diagnosis of PCOS can be made simply by a description of the symptoms. It may well be that no tests are necessary to make the diagnosis. For instance, for someone with unwanted hair growth in whom the interval between periods is greater than 5 weeks, then the diagnosis can be made with a high degree of certainty based on these features alone. There are very few other medical conditions that cause both irregular periods and hirsutism. Sometimes the full picture is not immediately obvious. Some women with PCOS may only have two periods per year and no sign of hirsutism while others might have extensive hirsutism with perfectly regular periods. An individual therefore can have any one or more of the symptoms.

Another way of looking at the variety of PCOS features is as a spectrum of symptoms with the severe end applying to those women with one or two periods per year as well as marked hirsutism and acne. The mild end of the spectrum includes women with regular cycles and slight hirsutism.

The ultrasound appearance of polycystic ovaries is a key factor used in making the diagnosis. The polycystic ovary is often slightly larger than average and contains more than twelve follicles on the ultrasound scan compared to smaller ovaries which contain fewer than 12 follicles and is defined as 'normal'.

In 2003 a group of experts met in Rotterdam in the Netherlands to agree on criteria for the diagnosis of PCOS. They came up with a consensus definition that is as follows:

Rotterdam criteria of the diagnosis of PCOS

A woman is considered to have PCOS if she has at least 2 of these features:

- Evidence of androgen excess either with symptoms such as hirsutism and acne, or with raised testosterone in the blood

- Irregular periods with intervals between periods extending greater than 35 days on occasion

- Polycystic ovaries on ultrasound

why is the diagnosis of PCOS sometimes missed?

While many women with PCOS may have the classical picture combining all 3 components of the Rotterdam criteria that make up the diagnosis, others may have less obvious symptoms or test results that are not clear-cut. With all of the symptoms it can sometimes be difficult to decide when one is truly outside of the expected range. For instance, is acne in a 17-year-old a normal part of adolescence or does it indicate PCOS? In the following section each of the symptoms are considered in turn to get an idea of how normal is defined. An exploration of each symptom group is covered in subsequent chapters.

irregular periods

Oligomenorrhoea is a term used to describe period intervals between 35 days and 6 months. This is the most common menstrual irregularity in PCOS. The term *amenorrhoea* is used when there has been no period for at least 6 months and while this can often be part of PCOS, there is a long list of other conditions that can also cause this.

It is generally accepted that the length of a normal menstrual cycle may vary between 25 and 35 days. The phrase *irregular periods* is ambiguous because it can mean different things to different people. It might be applied to someone who has one short cycle 26 days long followed by one that is 34 days long even though both are right at the margin of what might be accepted as normal variability. Periods may also be irregular in their flow by being very light one month but very heavy the next. This pattern of variable flow is not a key feature of PCOS – it is the timing between periods that is the key feature. Other menstrual problems such as excessive pain during a period or mood swings in the premenstrual week are not specific to PCOS.

hirsutism and acne

Hirsutism is a term applied to unwanted hair growth affecting various parts of the body beyond those that are expected for the average female. The common places for hair growth to be a problem are on the face and the abdomen from the pubic area to the tummy button. The arms and legs and back can also be affected in some women. Hirsutism is a sign of too much testosterone being made and PCOS is by far the most common cause of this problem. There are many treatments available for hirsutism and usually a combination can be found that will be effective. Unfortunately, it is rare to find a simple treatment that makes the problem go away forever.

Acne is a common problem during the teenage years and only a minority of adolescents with acne will be found to have PCOS. Acne that persists into the 20s however, is more unusual and can be a key feature of PCOS. Indeed, acne can be the only significant symptom. As both acne and irregular periods are common in young adolescents, a certain diagnosis of PCOS is often not made with certainty until several years have passed.

how did they work out what a polycystic ovary looked like with ultrasound?

Even though ultrasound scanning of the ovary is a key part of the diagnosis of PCOS, getting a good picture is not always straightforward. It is useful to cover a little background of how ultrasound of the ovary has developed over the years.

Ultrasound machines began to be useful for looking at the ovary in the early 1980s. This was the time when the resolution of ultrasound pictures was advanced enough to clearly identify the follicles within the ovary in order to allow for accurate counting. Ultrasound was first used to observe how the follicles matured and how the dominant follicle finally developed in women who were trying to conceive. It was noted that a proportion of women who were receiving fertility treatment had a tendency to develop many follicles, whereas other women consistently developed only a single dominant follicle. This was an important issue as those with several follicles would be at risk of developing twins or even triplets or more.

After observing the differences in how the ovaries behaved during fertility treatment, it was soon realised that those women who usually produced a single follicle tended to have fewer than 10 visible follicles at the start of treatment while those that had a tendency to produce a lot of follicles started with more than 10 small ones at the outset. Also, those women with greater than 10 follicles included some with clear-cut symptoms such as irregular periods and unwanted hair growth.

The advent of good quality ultrasound in the 1980s therefore, widened the spectrum of women included as having PCOS based on the number of follicles in the resting ovary instead of just blood tests. The cut-off point of 10 follicles each between 2 and 10 mm was established using an ultrasound probe on the outside of the abdomen and looking through to the ovaries after the bladder has been filled. The full bladder was important to push aside the neighboring bowels and to gain a clear picture of the ovaries.

Another ultrasound probe was then developed that could be inserted into the vagina and close to the ovaries which gave a much better close-up picture. For women who have been sexually active therefore, a change was made from trans-abdominal to trans-vaginal ultrasound whenever possible. Because of the greater resolution that is achieved using vaginal scans, it was agreed that the cut-off point between normal ovaries and polycystic ovaries based on follicle number would then be 12.

It must be noted however, that a single cut-off point such as 12 follicles is arbitrary and that there will be a grey area surrounding this magic number 12. There may be some months when slightly fewer follicles become active and only 10 follicles can be seen, whereas in other months by random chance 13 follicles may be active. In other words, the body is not precise enough to behave in exactly the same way every month.

It is very easy for even an inexperienced ultrasound technician to identify a clear-cut polycystic ovary that is enlarged with many obvious follicles. This is commonly the picture in women with very infrequent periods. In those women with hirsutism but regular periods the ultrasound appearance can be more subtle. The ovaries may not be enlarged and the very small follicles can be hard to see, and so it might take a specialist in ovary ultrasound to patiently count all of the follicles in both ovaries.

how do you get a good ultrasound picture?

The most common problem with ultrasound is to miss a subtle version of polycystic ovaries – a false negative scan.

Ultrasound is very much in the eye of the beholder, so much so that even when using exactly the same machine, two people scanning may arrive at slightly different conclusions. Those who are scanning as part of fertility treatment gain an enormous experience of the varying picture within the ovary. Those scanners who may be looking at the liver, the kidney or the ovary depending on the day may miss some subtle differences. Within the ovary it is easy to miss the very small follicles between 2 and 5 mm.

At the time of ovulation the dominant follicle can be almost half of the size of the ovary. This makes it very difficult to read the detail in the ovary that is squashed to one side. Similarly, after ovulation the corpus luteum will also distort the adjacent ovary tissue. For this reason the best ultrasound picture is obtained in the first week of the cycle even before the period has stopped. This is a time when neither ovary is distorted by large follicles allowing both to be read with clarity.

In young women who have not been sexually active, a trans-abdominal ultrasound is required instead of a trans-vaginal scan. Sometimes in this situation a low-fibre diet should be followed for 3 days prior to the scan to try to clear gas within the intestines which can get in the way of a clear picture. Also, at the time of the scan you have to drink a lot of water to fill the bladder which form a clear 'window' through which to view the ovaries.

what about 3D, 4D and magnetic resonance scanning?

The technology of ultrasound scanning is constantly improving. Think of the difference between the appearance of a television screen in the 1980s compared to the high definition screens currently available. As ultrasound improves, so the ability to detect smaller follicles in the ovary becomes more accurate. It is likely that the criterion of 12 follicles for the diagnosis of polycystic ovaries may change.

All routine scans of the ovary are made in two dimensions. With two-dimensional (2D) scanning several passes have to be made through the ovary to make sure that all follicles are identified. With three-dimensional (3D) scanning, the ovary is scanned three times, once in each plane perpendicular to each other. A computer then reconstructs a 3D image and each follicle can then be counted. Four-dimensional (4D) scanning is a recent advance on 3D where the computer is faster so that the image appears in real time – the fourth dimension is time. 3D and 4D scanning are useful tools and may well become more available but for now they are used mainly in research.

Magnetic resonance imaging or MRI is often thought to be a gold standard of scanning but in fact for the ovary, ultrasound is much more useful.

how can the diagnosis of PCOS be made in error?

Because there is no single test that clinches the diagnosis of PCOS the label can be applied wrongly. Remember, the ultrasound appearance of a polycystic ovary occurs in 20% of all women. There is always a possibility therefore, that the ultrasound part of the diagnosis occurs by chance and that there is another reason for the symptoms. The most common situation when this occurs is in women with amenorrhoea. According to the Rotterdam criteria a woman with amenorrhoea and polycystic ovaries qualifies for the diagnosis of PCOS, but of course there are other reasons for lack of periods and the ultrasound appearance of polycystic ovaries may be an incidental finding. The time to be alert that the diagnosis of PCOS is not secure is in women *without* hirsutism.

One common situation where periods can stop is in women who are either losing weight, are slightly underweight or take more than the average amount of exercise. Weight loss can cause a switch-off of the drive to the pituitary gland that in turn drives the ovary. This is called hypothalamic amenorrhoea. The hormone levels on the blood test can often be normal just as they are in PCOS. Sometimes the ultrasound picture can look very similar to polycystic ovaries if no ovulation is occurring. The ovary appearance in hypothalamic amenorrhoea is often described as *multicystic* rather than polycystic and the subtle differences between the two are hard to spot.

There are several conditions that cause hirsutism that can be confused with PCOS. These conditions are relatively rare. Testosterone is also made by the adrenal glands and there is an inherited condition where this is made in excess. This condition is called late onset congenital adrenal hyperplasia. It accounts for less than one in 100 women with hirsutism. Some centres routinely screen for this condition by measuring a particular marker in the blood – 17-hydroxyprogesterone. Other centres will only test for this if the level of testosterone is very high. Although there are other causes for hirsutism they rarely cause confusion because they occur quite suddenly and grow worse over a matter of weeks. This sudden onset is typical of nodules within the ovary or adrenal gland that make testosterone whereas the pattern in PCOS is of a very gradual onset over a matter of months.

making the diagnosis in teenagers

The symptoms of PCOS commonly start during adolescence soon after the first period. At this time in life however, irregular periods and acne are common in their own right and therefore the diagnosis of PCOS in this age group is often brought into question. It is usually accepted that irregular periods should have settled down within one year of the start of menstruation and so if irregular periods persist for 2 to 3 years then the possibility of PCOS arises. However, one should be cautious about making the diagnosis of PCOS in teenage years. It is always worth reassessing in the early 20s to see how many of the symptoms go away on their own. This is particularly so if early treatment with a combined oral contraceptive has masked the ability to read symptoms accurately. It can be a good idea to interrupt the pill for some months in order to undertake a reassessment.

Adolescence is a time when the ovaries are working at their highest level in life and this may explain why symptoms are more prominent in this age group. In addition, towards the end of the growth spurt there is a natural, physiological insulin resistance that gradually subsides over later teenage years. Therefore, some of the symptoms of PCOS may get better between the ages of 18 and 22. Also, because of this insulin resistance of adolescence, some doctors feel that metformin is particularly effective in this age group compared to its use in older women.

if blood tests are not essential for the diagnosis, how are they useful?

For many women with clear-cut symptoms, a blood test is not essential to make the diagnosis of PCOS. The main reason for doing blood tests is to exclude other causes of irregular periods and hirsutism. The results from blood tests are often entirely normal and this can be reassuring. The hallmark features of PCOS on a blood test are raised measurements of the hormones LH and testosterone. The concentration of LH in the blood tends to be high in women who have very irregular periods whereas testosterone concentrations tend to be high in women with severe hirsutism.

The reason why not too much emphasis is placed on the blood test results is that the measurements can be very variable. Different testosterone results from blood samples taken from one person may be different depending on the time of day or day of the month. The hormone LH rises to a high peak at the time of ovulation and so blood tests taken in the middle of a regular cycle may well show a high LH level for this reason. In addition, the levels of LH within the blood are pulsatile meaning that they rise and fall every 90 minutes. It is this pulsatility that transmits most of the detailed information to the ovary to signal the growth of a follicle.

The measurement of testosterone is subject to a great deal of variation because of technical problems in the laboratory. Some researchers have argued that the measurement of testosterone is so variable that it is not a useful measurement in women at all. Having said this, measurements of testosterone are important for women with severe hirsutism and if the levels are particularly high, then more detailed tests of the adrenal gland might be needed.

In the next section on blood tests, other hormones such as insulin, thyroxine and prolactin are considered in more detail.

what blood tests might be considered for a woman with PCOS?

For many women with PCOS a blood test may not be absolutely necessary. In this section the common blood test requests are listed first. More unusual blood tests are listed after, together with the reasons why they might be requested.

Hormone Reference Table

A brief reference table of hormones that are relevant to PCOS. Remember that it is rarely necessary to measure most of these. Laboratory methods vary a lot and are therefore the reference range is only a guide to the two common ways of reporting results

Hormone	where it is made	what the hormone does	importance in PCOS	reference range UK (non-UK)
17 hydroxy – progesterone (17OHP)	adrenal gland and corpus luteum	this is a marker for congenital adrenal hyperplasia which is a form of testosterone excess from the adrenal gland	can be slightly raised and should be tested if testosterone is exceptionally high	1-6 nmol/L (50-350 ng/dL)
Androstenedione (A4)	adrenal gland and ovary	a week anti-androgen which is the step before turning into testosterone	usually reads exactly the same as testosterone and therefore is rarely required	2.6-7.2 nmol/L (75-200 ng/dL)
Anti-Müllerian hormone (AMH)	Ovary follicles	made by small follicles in the ovary and may control follicle selection	can be raised in proportion to how many follicles are seen	20-70 pmol/L (3-10 ng/mL)
Dehydroepi-androsterone (DHEAS)	adrenal gland and to a lesser extent the ovary	this is a weak form of testosterone and is the step before making androstenedione	some women make predominantly DHEAS instead of testosterone but measuring DHEAS is not usually required	2-12 umol/L (50-450 ug/dL)
Follicle stimulating hormone (FSH)	pituitary gland	drives the conversion of testosterone to oestrogen	usually normal in PCOS, if raised can be a marker for low ovarian reserve	2-10 mu/L (2-10 miu/mL)
Insulin	pancreas	is essential for controlling glucose levels	although it can be raised it is not usually useful to measure insulin	10-60 pmol/L (2-20 mu/L)

Hormone	Source	Function	Notes	Values
Luteinising hormone (LH)	pituitary gland	drives the ovary to make testosterone, also triggers ovulation	Often raised particularly in women with irregular periods and who are not overweight	2-10 mU/L (2-10 mu/L)
Oestradiol	ovary	for fertility oestrogen is important to prepare the womb lining in the first 2 weeks of the cycle	usually normal in PCOS but can be useful to measure in women with amenorrhoea	100-1600 pmol/L (30-400 pg/mL)
Progesterone	corpus luteum	essential for preparing the womb lining for implantation of an embryo in the second 2 weeks of the cycle	can be used to check if ovulation has occurred with a blood test one week later	To confirm ovulation: >25 nmol/L (>10 ng/mL)
Prolactin	pituitary gland	prepares the body for breastfeeding, goes up in stress and commonly fluctuates.	raised in 10% of women with PCOS and can cause amenorrhoea when raised threefold	80-490 uIU/mL (4-22 ug/L)
Sex hormone binding globulin (SHBG)	liver	carries testosterone and oestrogen in the blood. A useful marker of insulin resistance and overweight where it reads low	can be used to assess insulin resistance and response to treatment or weight loss	15-75 nmol/L (0.5-3.5 ug/dL)
Testosterone	adrenal gland and ovary	is made in all women and is necessary to make oestrogen	can be raised but is commonly normal	0.1-1.8 nmol/L (10-60 ng/dL)
Thyroid-stimulating hormone (TSH)	pituitary gland	controls the thyroid gland to make thyroxine	not critical to PCOS but is often included on routine testing	0.3-4.2 mU/L (0.3 – 4.2 mU/L)
Thyroxine (Free T4)	thyroid gland	controls the metabolic rate of the body	not critical to PCOS but is often included on routine testing	12-22 pmol/L (0.9-2.3 ng/mL)

luteinising hormone (LH)

LH, together with FSH, are the two fertility hormones made by the pituitary gland. Collectively they are called gonadotrophins. LH drives the cells surrounding each follicle to make testosterone and FSH in turn drives the follicle cells to convert testosterone to oestrogen. It is normal therefore, for all women to make testosterone as part of the pathway to making oestrogen.

LH reaches a peak at the time of ovulation and takes part in triggering the release of the egg from the mature follicle. It is LH that appears in the urine and can be measured with ovulation testing kits. In the second half of the cycle LH drives the corpus luteum to make progesterone which prepares the lining of the womb for the embryo.

The normal range for LH is between 2 and 12 mu/L and most commonly the level is similar to that of FSH somewhere in the middle of the reference range in women with PCOS. LH measurements can rise to fivefold higher than average particularly in the first phase of the cycle or permanently for women with amenorrhoea.

Some textbooks emphasise the ratio between LH and FSH as being important. When the LH:FSH ratio is greater than 2 it was said to be diagnostic of PCOS. In fact, this ratio can vary quite a lot in women with PCOS so this rule is not very useful. For instance, if the blood sample is taken a little late in the cycle when the LH level rises to trigger ovulation then the LH:FSH ratio is often above 2. Apart from this confusion, when a sample is taken at the time of ovulation, a raised LH measurement is a good marker for PCOS and occurs in very few other conditions. On the other hand, LH measurements are completely normal in approximately two thirds of women with PCOS.

follicle-stimulating hormone (FSH)

Measurements of FSH are usually normal in women with PCOS. The main reason for measuring FSH is to give a background assessment of the health of the ovary and how many eggs there are left. As a woman approaches the menopause the levels of FSH in the blood gradually rise from the usual 2 – 10 mu/L to be greater than 50 mu/L. Therefore, when the FSH measurement rises towards the upper border of the normal range it is likely that the number of eggs left within the ovary is declining and that the chances of achieving a pregnancy are reduced.

testosterone

Testosterone is made by cells called theca cells that surround each follicle. In the follicle, testosterone then passes through to the inner layer of granulosa cells where it is converted to oestrogen. Theca cells from women with PCOS have a natural tendency to make more testosterone than average. This effect is seen even when the cells are removed from the body and put into a test tube. Apart from the ovary, the only other gland in the body that makes testosterone is the adrenal gland. On blood testing, the level of testosterone is often normal in women with PCOS and the main reason to measure it is to rule out other rare causes of testosterone excess which tend to give very high readings.

Every laboratory gives a slightly different reference range for testosterone which is commonly given as 0.2 to 1.8 nmol/L. Results greater than 5 nmol/L would be considered sufficiently high to warrant further exploration before concluding that PCOS was the cause of the problem.

Testosterone is carried in the bloodstream attached to a protein called sex hormone binding globulin or SHBG. So when you read a testosterone result, the laboratory has actually measured both testosterone and SHBG together.

In fact, 95% of testosterone when measured on a blood test is bound to proteins and it is only the 5% of free testosterone that is important in causing acne and hirsutism. Measurement of that 5% of free testosterone is technically very difficult and inaccurate, and so we make do with total testosterone measurements on the whole.

Measurements of testosterone can be easily affected by conditions that alter SHBG. The most common of these conditions is overweight which results in lower SHBG concentrations and therefore an under-estimate of the impact of testosterone. Many blood result printouts will automatically print a fudge factor to account for the effect of SHBG which is called the free androgen index or FAI (FAI = [testosterone x SHBG] divided by 100). This is a very crude correction equation that some doctors find useful.

Testosterone is notoriously difficult to measure in a consistent fashion not only because of the very small amounts that circulate in women but also because of technical difficulties in measuring this type of hormone using automated laboratory methods. In many ways a woman's symptoms are a more sensitive method of determining the impact of testosterone than a blood measurement.

sex hormone binding globulin (SHBG)

SHBG is a carrier protein that is bound to testosterone and oestrogen in the bloodstream.

SHBG concentrations are very closely related to body weight. In someone who is overweight SHBG levels are low but they increase with weight loss. The hormone insulin is the link that connects bodyweight to SHBG production. At a higher body weight, the circulating levels of insulin are raised and this hormone switches off the production of SHBG. In this way, SHBG can be used as a simple method of determining how sensitive the body is to insulin or in other words the state of *insulin resistance*.

Since bodyweight is so closely related to SHBG it might be said that measuring weight is a more cost-effective test than measuring SHBG!

prolactin

Prolactin is a hormone made by the pituitary gland in specific cells alongside those making LH and FSH. The only important role of prolactin is during pregnancy to prepare a woman for breastfeeding. Very high prolactin levels can cause leakage of breast milk which is called *galactorrhoea*. It is rare for women with PCOS to get this symptom because the levels of prolactin are usually normal or only moderately raised. Prolactin can be made by a nodule within the pituitary gland called a prolactinoma or alternatively prolactin excess can be caused by some tablet treatments particularly those in the anti-sickness family. When prolactin runs high the body is fooled into thinking that the woman is breastfeeding and so the pituitary gland in turn switches off LH and FSH causing a lack of periods, just as would occur in a woman who is breastfeeding. The measurement of prolactin is therefore always on the list for women with irregular periods.

A modest rise in prolactin occurs in approximately 10% of women with PCOS, probably reflecting the altered hormone pattern coming from the ovary. There are specific tablets that switch off the production of prolactin from the pituitary gland. These are occasionally advised for women with PCOS.

androstenedione and DHEAS

DHEAS and androstenedione are in the chemical pathway that leads to testosterone. In any situation where testosterone may be raised, these two hormones may also be high. There is no particular value in measuring all three of these and therefore testing for DHEAS or androstenedione is not usually necessary. Some textbooks refer to DHEAS as an indicator of testosterone coming from the adrenal glands but in fact this rule often does not apply.

DHEAS is raised in approximately 10% of women with PCOS and contributes to unwanted hair growth. DHEAS levels return to normal with treatment that includes the combined oral contraceptive pill. This indicates that in this situation, the origin of the hormone is the ovary and not the adrenal gland as stated in some textbooks.

Together, these three hormones are called *androgens*. As they often all three rise together, the term *androgen excess* or *hyperandrogenism* is used instead of testosterone excess. Similarly, we use the term *anti-androgens* instead of testosterone blockers.

fasting glucose and insulin

Fasting glucose and insulin measurements can be used to determine how effective insulin is in the body, or, in other words, the level of insulin resistance. While this is an important topic in research, in everyday practice measurements of fasting glucose and insulin are not very revealing. Most guidelines state that insulin measurements are not required as part of investigations in PCOS. Fasting glucose measurements are not a very sensitive method of detecting risk of diabetes and therefore if there is a suspicion of diabetes then an oral glucose tolerance test is much more sensitive.

oral glucose tolerance test (OGTT)

An oral glucose tolerance test is the gold standard method of diagnosing diabetes and detecting a risk of future diabetes. The test starts with an overnight fast and the first blood test is taken before drinking a standard 75 g glucose drink. Between 2 and 4 further blood tests are taken over the next two hours. Plasma glucose measurements are made on every blood sample. In this way it can be seen how the body handles glucose. If the body is not very efficient at disposing of glucose then higher than average levels are seen over the two hours of the test. The most important time-point for which there are reference points for diabetes risk is at 2 hours.

An OGTT should be considered in the following circumstances:

* If there is a parent with type 2 diabetes

* Previous diabetes in pregnancy

* Body mass index greater than 35 kg/m²

* Symptoms of diabetes such as thirst or passing urine often

How to diagnose diabetes based on fasting glucose or OGTT result		
	Fasting blood glucose (mmol/L)	2 Hour OGTT result
Normal	<6.1	<7.8
Impaired fasting glucose	6.1–6.9	
Impaired glucose tolerance		7.8–11.1
Diabetes	>11.1	>11.1

cholesterol profile

A cholesterol profile is a group of results that make up most of the types of cholesterol in the blood. Usually included

examples of oral glucose tolerance test results

A glucose drink is taken at time 0 and then blood samples are drawn to measure how glucose is handled by the body. Sometimes samples are taken only at 0 and 120 minutes as these are the vital times for diagnosis.

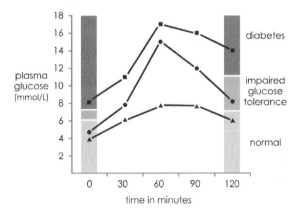

are these four results: total cholesterol, triglycerides, HDL-cholesterol and LDL-cholesterol. This test is usually requested for people with a risk of heart disease. The risk of heart disease in PCOS is a hotly debated topic. In fact there is very little direct evidence that heart disease is a problem in PCOS and so a cholesterol profile is not really required.

For women who might be at risk of diabetes however, the cholesterol profile is interesting because of a particular fingerprint indicating insulin resistance. In women with insulin resistance triglycerides are typically raised and HDL-cholesterol reads low.

thyroid function test – free thyroxine (free T4) and TSH

An imbalance of thyroid hormone commonly causes irregular periods and can contribute to weight gain. Because these are both features of PCOS, thyroid function tests are almost always included in the investigation of PCOS. Thyroid function tests usually include measurements of the hormone that is made by the thyroid gland – *thyroxine* – together with the thyroid-regulating hormone from the pituitary gland – *thyroid stimulating hormone* or TSH. The most common association with PCOS is an underactive thyroid gland where the free thyroxine measurement may be low or low normal and more importantly the TSH measurement is raised (it goes in the opposite direction).

adrenal gland tests – 17-hydroxyprogesterone, synacthen test and cortisol

Tests for the adrenal gland may be needed if the testosterone level has been found to be very high or if the degree of unwanted hair is at the severe end of the spectrum for PCOS. The most common condition of the adrenal gland that can mimic PCOS is late onset or non-classical congenital adrenal hyperplasia. This is a condition where there is a mild resistance to the production of the main adrenal hormone *cortisol* within the adrenal gland. As a result, the adrenal gland makes too much testosterone. The chemical fingerprint that can be found in the blood in this condition is a compound called 17-hydroxyprogesterone which can either be measured as a single test or as part of a stimulation test for the adrenal gland – a Synacthen test.

A Synacthen test should be performed in the morning and requires no particular preparation. Blood tests are taken before and after an injection of Synacthen which is a synthetic hormone that stimulates the adrenal gland. Two to three blood samples are taken in total over 30 to 60 min. A measurement of 17-hydroxyprogesterone greater than 30 nmol/L makes the diagnosis of CAH. In this condition there are other treatment options and this is particularly important if infertility is part of the picture.

The adrenal gland makes the hormone cortisol and if too much is made then a rare condition called Cushing's syndrome is the result. Cushing's syndrome shares some of the features of PCOS including overweight and hirsutism which is why tests for this condition are sometimes requested. The two most common tests are a 24-hour urine collection for cortisol and a blood test also for cortisol that is taken at 9 am in the morning after taking tablets of a synthetic steroid called dexamethasone at 10 pm the night before. This test is called an overnight dexamethasone suppression test.

anti-müllerian hormone (AMH)

AMH has arrived on the scene relatively recently and its main purpose is to estimate how many follicles remain within the ovary as it grows older. AMH is made in the ovary by the small to medium sized follicles. As the numbers of follicles decline with age so too does the measurement of AMH reaching a low level after the menopause. As women with PCOS have more than the average number of follicles, the concentration of AMH in the circulation is often raised. The levels of AMH are about 2-fold higher in PCOS compared to women with normal ovaries.

AMH generally remains within the realm of research and is not commonly used for routine purposes in many clinics focusing on PCOS. While levels can be higher in PCOS than average, there is a great deal of overlap with the normal range and so this is not a particularly useful diagnostic test. As AMH measurements becomes more available however, we are likely to find that they can be useful in many situations when the diagnosis of PCOS may be in doubt.

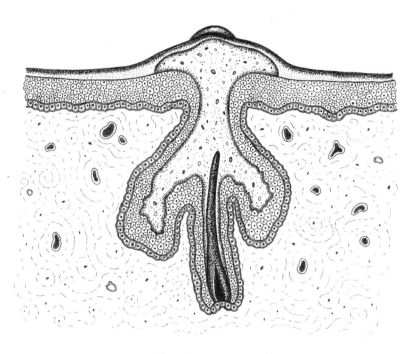

pilosebaceous unit

This is a diagram of the surface of the skin focusing on a sebaceous gland that is forming an acne spot. The centre of the picture shows the skin grease or sebum being made by the gland with a spot of inflammation – a blackhead – at the top. Some sebaceous glands have a hair follicle. This is shown at the bottom of the picture and the two together are called a pilosebaceous unit.

chapter 3
hirsutism, acne and alopecia

introduction

The skin covering the entire surface of the body is very sensitive to hormonal changes, particularly to the level of testosterone. The action of testosterone on the skin is the reason why men and women have different skin textures. Male skin tends to be courser and thicker compared to the female. The pattern of hair growth over the body is a clear sign of action of testosterone, which circulates in men at 10 times the level found in women. Hair is mainly made of the protein keratin.

Testosterone can also drive the sebaceous and sweat glands in the skin to work overtime, which causes clogging of the pores followed by inflammation and infection that is the basis for acne. Excess sweating can occur as part of PCOS but is not all that common. Sweating or 'hyperhydrosis' can also have other causes. Sebaceous glands make *seborrhoea* that is the technical name for skin grease. This is a common problem in PCOS that responds well to anti-androgen treatment.

In susceptible individuals, testosterone can switch off hair growth in scalp hair follicles. This leads to the distressing symptom of *alopecia* or scalp hair thinning. In contrast, testosterone switches <u>on</u> body hair growth on all other parts of the body especially face, tummy and legs. It is a mystery how testosterone can have two different effects on different parts of the body. Of the three common androgenic symptoms, acne tends to appear first followed by hirsutism and then some years later by alopecia (of course there are many times when this general rule is not followed). The response to anti-androgen treatment tends to be in the same sequence but in reverse, with acne improving over 8 to 12 weeks, hirsutism over 3 to 12 months and alopecia on an even longer timescale.

The level of testosterone in the blood is not very closely regulated in women. This is why androgen-related symptoms are so common. For instance, in the thyroid gland there is a very close regulation by the pituitary hormone TSH making sure that the level of thyroxine is held steady. There is no such system regulating testosterone in the body in women. Testosterone is therefore allowed to fluctuate, causing mischief on the skin surface when it runs high.

The skin is also sensitive to the hormone insulin but only when there are very high levels in the circulation. *Acanthosis nigricans* describes a band of dark skin around the base of the neck and also in the armpits that has a velvety nature to the touch. This skin change is a sign of insulin resistance and is most noticeable in women with a dark complexion and who are very overweight.

Hidradenitis suppurativa describes blocking of the sweat glands, often in the armpits and groin, to form abscesses and boils which can grow large enough to require surgery. Hidradenitis is more common in women with PCOS who are overweight and is treated in a similar way to acne.

hirsutism

the biology of hair growth

There are two main types of hair covering the body. Vellus hair is fine with no colour to it. This type of hair can be found on close inspection over most of the body, apart from the palms of the hands and the soles of the feet. Terminal hair is the thickened, darker hair. One action of testosterone is to convert the vellus hair to terminal hair. It is terminal hair that causes all of the problems in PCOS. It is thought that you cannot completely reverse the change from terminal to vellus hair but in fact you can reduce the growth pattern of terminal hair until its appearance is very difficult to distinguish from the vellus hair.

Terminal hair in the body grows in phases. Hair follicles are distributed randomly at different points of the growth cycle.

Anagen is the growth phase of hair that can last for anything between a few months and several years. Shorter hairs on the body, such as eyebrows, will grow for only a short time but the scalp hair, particularly in someone who can grow their hair down to the bottom of their back, may grow for up to 8 years. The average growth rate for hair is 1 cm per month and at any one time approximately 90% of hair follicles will be in the growth phase.

Catagen marks the end of growth where the hair follicles separate from the cells at the bottom of the follicle that produces their hair protein. Catagen lasts only a few weeks. Only about 1% of hair follicles will be in this phase.

Telogen is the resting phase for hair that lasts for a few months. As this phase comes to an end the hair is pushed out by new growth from a hair follicle beneath that is entering anagen. On average, about 10% of hair follicles are in this resting phase. The hair follicle however, is particularly vulnerable when it is in telogen. At times of stress, illness, vitamin or mineral deficiency or major hormone change then over 50% of follicles can enter telogen resulting in noticeable scalp hair fall out. This is called *telogen effluvium*. In addition, there is a seasonal shedding of hair which typically occurs in the winter months when more than the average number of hair follicles enter telogen phase. Soon after an event such as this hair should regrow if conditions are good.

the cycle of hair growth and fallout

An example of a 4-year growth cycle for hair follicles. Longer hair on the scalp may have a cycle length of several years. Having completed a cycle the follicle enters a rest phase before starting to grow again.

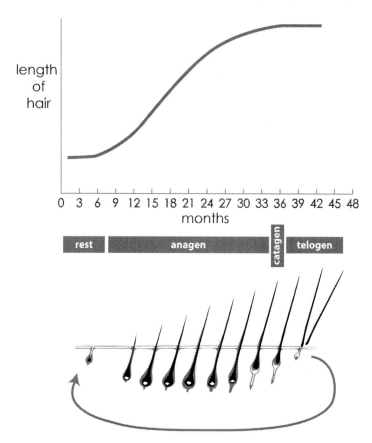

Treatments that block the action of testosterone act only in the growth phase to reduce the thickness of the hair follicle shaft and the speed of its growth. The reason why treatments for unwanted hair growth take so long to work is that you have to wait for sufficient numbers of follicles to have entered growth phase before they can be influenced by treatment. It can often take several months before enough follicles have gone through the stages of the cycle for a reduction in unwanted hair growth to be noticeable. Scalp hair fall-out therefore can be reduced if everything is in place to strengthen the hair follicle in telogen. This usually means topping up on vitamins and minerals that are known to stabilise the hair follicle.

how do you know if the amount of hair growth is more than average?

In order to decide whether the extent of unwanted hair growth is outside of the expected range, a scoring system was devised by counting the number of hairs in set regions of the body in a group of over 200 women who were all from a Caucasian background. A reference range was developed by two researchers who gave their name to the scoring system – the *Ferriman Gallwey* score (see chapter 11 for this reference). While this scoring system can be useful for research purposes it has its limitations for routine use in clinic. It does not take into account the differences between ethnic groups and not all doctors will count hairs in the same way. Also, women may not want to let hair grow to a natural level just to have a count performed. After all, it is how the person affected feels about the problem that matters, more than what the book says.

On the other hand, self-assessment of hair growth can be affected by low mood or the expectation of those around you. Depression can make the mind focus on hair growth as part of feeling low in self-confidence. Also, pictures of perfect women in advertisements bombard us all, where every blemish has been removed using Photoshop! These images change what is considered to be acceptable hair growth.

We have to accept that there is no scientific method of measuring the level of hair growth and it is seldom useful to make comparisons to an arbitrary normal range. A sensible balance has to be achieved between the impact of excess body hair on an individual and the measures that are taken to control it in terms of time, money and medical risk of drug treatment. The most common complaint from women with hirsutism is that a doctor has dismissed the problem as not being important enough to treat. The most common worry from doctors is that women may become so focused on the problem of excess hair growth that they may be willing to take unreasonable risks in order to control it. Hirsutism may not be life-threatening but nevertheless, it scores very highly amongst factors that affect self-confidence and quality-of-life.

does the hair growth pattern differ in different countries?

Some ethnic groups such as those from the Mediterranean or South Asian backgrounds experience more facial and body hair compared to Caucasian women. Oriental ethnic groups tend to have sparse unwanted hair growth but are said to be more prone to developing acne. It may be difficult for women to move from one country, where a certain amount of facial hair may be accepted, to another country, where they feel that the expectation from society is of lower amount of hair growth.

The underlying reason why different ethnic groups have a different pattern is not known. The explanation must lie buried in some detail of our genetic make up. A degree of variation occurs with the proportion of women who have polycystic ovaries in a population. It is thought that approximately 35% of women in Sri Lanka have polycystic ovaries compared to 20% in the UK. This may account for the higher number of women with hirsutism in South Asian populations. Another possible explanation for ethnic differences is in how sensitive hair is to the action of testosterone.

treatments for hirsutism

before taking any drug treatments, what are the options to control hirsutism?

Simple lifestyle measures can have a major beneficial effect on hirsutism. Most important of all is for women who are overweight to find an effective method of achieving weight loss. Excess weight causes insulin resistance which is a drive to the ovary to make testosterone. As weight comes off, so the testosterone levels in the circulation fall. This means that weight loss alone will improve unwanted hair growth although it can take some months for this benefit to be noticeable.

Weight loss also makes drug treatments more effective. One important lesson that was gained from a review of all of the studies of the treatment for hirsutism, was that women who were overweight always responded less well compared to women at a lower body weight.

I don't want to take any drugs for this – what can I do without taking tablets?

The first treatments that most people turn to are simple methods to remove hair from the skin surface such as waxing, shaving, plucking, threading and hair dissolving creams. These treatments can be effective for scattered hair growth or small areas. The points in favour of these treatments are that they are widely available and some are cheap. The downside of these treatments is that they are temporary – the unwanted hair can come back quite quickly. Hair removing creams are made of strong alkaline chemicals that break down the protein in hair and do not prevent hair growing again.

There is a commonly held belief that shaving may stimulate further hair growth but there is no scientific research to confirm this. Shaving does however, produce sharp cut ends to the hair which makes the hair seem worse than it may have been beforehand. As far as we know there is no signal from the outside skin surface to the cells that form hair at the bottom of each follicle to work harder.

electrolysis

Electrolysis has been used for many years. This is a method of destroying hair follicles by applying an electrical probe to each follicle one by one. A good feature about this treatment is that it is quite widely available and cheaper than its main competitor, laser treatment. On the down side, repeated treatments are necessary for dense areas of hair. There always seems to be another hair follicle nearby that can pick up growth after a neighbouring one has been treated.

laser hair removal

Laser treatment for hair growth has become increasingly popular as it is an efficient method of disrupting hair follicles over a wider area. The good thing about laser treatment is that when it is effective it can be really good. If you are lucky, laser can be the best option for providing long-lasting clearance of hair. Successful use of laser treatment may mean that fewer drug treatments are needed. The down side of laser treatment is that it is expensive and it does not suit every colouring. The treatment relies on there being a contrast between the colour of the hair and the colour of skin. For instance, the best effects can be seen in women with dark hair and light skin colour. Women with blonde hair or with dark skin are less amenable to treatment. With new types of laser treatment however, even women with very dark skin can achieve success. Another problem with laser treatment is that some skin types are prone to a slight sunburn-like reaction. If this occurs then the treatment cannot be used. At the first visit a test area is always treated so that the skin reaction can be assessed before treatment starts.

Laser treatment is usually offered on a monthly basis for six months. The idea behind this is that at each visit a new crop of hair follicles have gone into growth phase when they will be most sensitive to treatment. There seems to be a great deal of variation in the success rate from laser treatment. Some people experience a long-lasting suppression of hair growth while in others, the hair grows back quite quickly. There is no way of telling beforehand who will have a good response and one simply has to try a course of treatment to know whether it will be a good option for the long-term.

eflornithine (Vaniqa)

Eflornithine is a cream that is applied to the face twice per day. It is only available on prescription in the UK but some prescribers consider Vaniqa to be a cosmetic treatment so it is not always available on the NHS. This cream does not act like a commercial hair removal product. Instead, it penetrates the hair follicle and prevents the hair-producing cells from incorporating protein into the shaft of the hair. Eflornithine is only licensed for use on the face. It has to be used twice every day without fail in order to be successful. Clearance of hair takes about 12 weeks. Some people find that this treatment irritates the skin or causes ingrowing hairs, in which case it cannot be used. The treatment only works for the time it is applied and gradually wears off once treatment has stopped. Eflornithine can work very well in conjunction with laser treatment.

Eflornithine can be very effective at the time of the menopause when the drive to hirsutism is a little less. In this age group its use might mean that no tablet treatment is required which is a great benefit. Another important feature of this treatment is that it works more quickly than tablet treatments. Therefore, a useful way of using this cream is to start at the same time as tablet treatment and then continue for three months. From then on, the tablet treatment might begin to take hold. This strategy is particularly useful for young women who are acutely distressed by unwanted hair growth and would benefit from a rapid response.

what about tablet treatments?

Tablet treatments work in two ways – by suppressing the amount of testosterone made by the ovary or by blocking the action of testosterone on the hair cells. Tablet treatment is commonly used when surface treatments have been exhausted or when there are two problems relating to testosterone. For instance, if acne and hirsutism occur together then the best option is to use a tablet treatment that will improve both symptoms. Similarly, if hirsutism is extensive then it is simply impossible for surface treatments alone to cope with the problem.

combined oral contraceptive pills (COCP)

Often the first type of treatment to be considered for PCOS is the combined birth control pill. Combined pills contain both oestrogen (ethinylestradiol) and progesterone. Contraceptive pills that contain only progesterone – the mini pill or progesterone-only pill – are not effective treatments for hirsutism. The reason for this is that it is the oestrogen component that does most of the work.

Oestrogen in the pill is sensed by the pituitary gland which responds by shutting down the production of LH and FSH because the body no longer needs to make its own oestrogen. As a consequence, the drive to the ovary is switched off and the ovary goes quiet. The follicles in the ovary stop maturing so that no ovulation occurs – this is how the pill works as a contraceptive. At the same time, the amount of testosterone made by the ovary is almost completely switched off so that the blood levels of testosterone drop by about half (the adrenal gland continues to make some testosterone). Another beneficial effect of the combined pill is to increase the amount of SHBG which is made by the liver. This has the effect of 'mopping up' excess testosterone in the circulation preventing it from latching onto hair follicles.

Combined pills come in three strengths depending on the amount of ethinylestradiol in it: 35, 30 and 20 micrograms. In general, the higher-dose pills are more effective at controlling periods and probably also hair growth, but tend to have more side-effects. The lower-dose pills have fewer side effects but can be less effective at period control. At the beginning of treatment for severe hirsutism it is common to use one of the stronger pills. The plan would then be to gradually move down the scale to a lower-dose pill as the unwanted hair growth comes under control. As a general principle, the lowest dose of treatment that keeps the problem at bay is the best option.

Combined pills also differ in the type of progestogen in their make-up. Some pills contain a progestogen with slight 'testosterone-like' effect which might show itself as worsening acne. An example of this type of progestogen is norethisterone. These pills, often called second generation pills, are generally not advised for use in women who already have testosterone-based symptoms such as acne or hirsutism. Another group of pills – third generation – have a progestogen which has almost no testosterone-like effect and are considered neutral. The progestogens in this group include Gestoden, Desogestrel and Norgestimate. These pills are a good option for women with hirsutism and acne.

There are two further types of combined pill in which the progestogen has a slight 'anti-testosterone' or testosterone-blocking activity. Dianette and Yasmin are marketed specifically for acne and hirsutism because they have anti-androgenic forms of progestogen. The progestogens in this group include cyproterone and drosperinone. While these pills are very effective, there have been few trials comparing them to the 'neutral' family which can also be effective in their own right. Side effects such as low mood and weight gain are particularly common with Dianette and the use of

Yasmin can be restricted as it is one of the most expensive forms of oral contraception. These pills rank higher than most in the risk of a blood clot.

All combined contraceptive pills have side effects and these can sometimes develop even after taking them for some years. If in doubt, it is always worth trying two or three months off the pill to test how one feels. Headaches, mood swings and weight gain are all common experiences that might tempt you to stop the pill altogether or to try a lower-dose alternative.

The birth control pills are certainly not for everyone, not only because of side effects but also because of the risks of using them. One hidden risk behind the pill is of a blood clot or *thrombosis*. A thrombosis commonly occurs in the calf muscle that then becomes swollen and painful. Very rarely a blood clot can move to the lung to cause pain and breathlessness. The combined pills increase the risk of a thrombosis by at least a factor of 3. In many women who are fit and healthy with no risk factors, the risk of thrombosis is so low that the increase of a factor of 3 still does not amount to a great worry. If however, the background risk of thrombosis is already raised, such as it is in smokers and anyone overweight, then the combined pills should not be used. Other contraindications to the combined pill are migraine headaches and high blood pressure. This is why the blood pressure should be checked every six months when taking the pill. One further worry for women who use the pill for many years is that the risk of breast cancer can be slightly increased later in life. All of these issues have to be taken into account when a prescription for the pill is started or renewed.

anti-androgens

Anti-androgens or testosterone-blockers work in two ways. They either block the testosterone receptor on the hair follicle or they stop testosterone being turned into its more potent cousin *dihydrotestosterone*.

how anti-androgen treatments work

How the anti-androgens (A) and the pill (B) work. With anti-androgens everything works normally but testosterone is blocked from acting on the hair follicle. The pill switches off the pituitary from making LH and FSH reducing the drive to the ovary and the amount of testosterone being made.

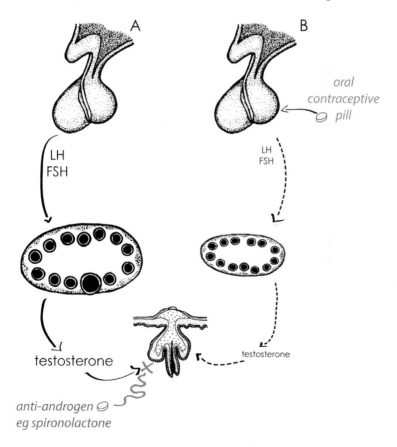

Testosterone receptor-blockers are the most commonly used anti-androgens. They are also called competitive antagonists. This means that they occupy the space on the hair follicle that testosterone would usually latch onto to do its work – the *androgen receptor*. In this way, testosterone bypasses the hair follicle which remains happily quiet. This group includes cyproterone acetate, spironolactone and flutamide.

The second group of anti-androgens block the conversion of testosterone to dihydrotestosterone, a step that is carried out by an enzyme in the skin called *5-alpha reductase*. Members of this family include finasteride and dutasteride. This group of anti-androgens were mainly developed for use in men with prostate cancer and are not marketed for use in women in the UK. There is however, a large body of research evidence showing the effectiveness of this type of treatment in women, mainly for alopecia but also for hirsutism.

Cyproterone acetate has been the most widely used anti-androgen in PCOS in the past. It is generally used in conjunction with an oral contraceptive pill, because on its own it acts to stop periods altogether as oestrogen is also switched off. Cyproterone is given for up to 10 days of each calendar month, usually for the first 10 days of each pack of the pill. The dose range is between 25 and 100 mg daily but because the higher doses tend to produce more side effects, a single 50 mg tablet for 10 days each month is usually the best starting point. Side effects to cyproterone include headache, depression and weight gain and these are sufficiently common to make this form of treatment less popular in recent years. At a very high dose, cyproterone acetate has been shown to have a bad effect on the liver and therefore a blood test for liver enzymes should take place every six months during use.

Spironolactone is very commonly used in PCOS for the treatment of acne and hirsutism. This treatment comes from a family of water tablets, or diuretics, although the effect on passing urine is barely noticeable in most women. Spironolactone has a completely separate use in people with heart failure where the diuretic property is important. In young women, it is the anti-androgen property of this drug that is the most prominent.

The dose range for spironolactone is between 25 and 200 mg daily taken either once per day or split into two doses. The higher dose range brings about the greatest side effects of which breakthrough menstrual bleeding is the most common problem. The side effects of spironolactone come about because it has oestrogen-like activity and this causes heavier periods or unscheduled breakthrough bleeding anywhere in the cycle. This side effect can improve if the dose is reduced but for some women it means that this treatment cannot be used conveniently. If this treatment is combined with a contraceptive pill then the period pattern is not commonly a problem. The great value of spironolactone is that, unlike cyproterone, it does not need to be combined with the pill and so can be used in smokers or overweight women on its own or with a progesterone-only pill such as Cerazette. Some prescribers are worried about using an anti-androgen without contraceptive cover because they fear the possibility of exposing pregnant women to these drugs.

Flutamide is the most rarely used anti-androgen because it is the most problematic for liver function. Flutamide can cause a drug-induced hepatitis on rare occasions and therefore regular monitoring of liver enzymes on blood testing is required. Flutamide however, is probably the most potent of the anti-androgens used in PCOS and so might be considered in exceptional situations.

Finasteride is the most common member of the family of inhibitors of 5 alpha reductase prescribed for women with PCOS. There are a few anecdotal reports of its cousin dutasteride also being used for alopecia. Finasteride is generally very well tolerated and has few side effects. The main worry with this treatment is that it appears to be the most dangerous of all anti-androgens when used in pregnancy by mistake. Finasteride has the potential to make a male fetus develop with abnormalities and so if an unexpected pregnancy occurs then a termination is always recommended. Usual doses of finasteride in women are between 1 and 2.5 mg.

does metformin work for reducing unwanted hair growth?

Compared to the oral contraceptive pills and anti-androgens, metformin has only a small effect at reducing unwanted hair growth. Having said this, there are some situations where metformin can be an important part of the treatment plan.

Metformin is classified as an *insulin sensitiser*. This means that it makes the action of insulin in the body more efficient at controlling glucose. The body responds by making less insulin and so the level in the blood circulation drops by about 20% or 30%. The lower insulin level reduces the drive to the ovary to make testosterone and so the testosterone levels also fall. This drop in testosterone, however, is not as much as you can get from using the pill. Nevertheless, several research studies have shown that hirsutism improves after treatment with metformin.

Metformin is particularly helpful in situations where the combined oral contraceptive cannot be used – in particular in women who are overweight. The reason for this is that some women find that metformin helps with weight loss and this in itself will improve hair growth.

Most studies using metformin for hirsutism have used a standard dose of 1500 mg per day in divided doses – 500 mg three times a day after each meal. Metformin is more effective when combined with a low-carbohydrate diet and cardiovascular exercise which are two other ways of reducing insulin resistance. Depending on the response, the full dose of metformin is likely to continue for at least one year. Because the effect of metformin on hirsutism is not very strong, it is commonly combined with spironolactone that is an anti-androgen that can also be taken without the pill.

what happens to treatment in the long-term?

If alopecia or hirsutism is particularly resistant to treatment then it is possible to combine components from different groups. For instance, anti-androgens are commonly combined with an oral contraceptive pill. If these two treatments together are not sufficient then it is also possible to add finasteride. Often, it is effective to use a low dose of two anti-androgens rather than a high dose of any single agent. It is not recommended that spironolactone and cyproterone be combined as we have no knowledge of how they may behave together.

All tablet treatments for hirsutism tend to wear off when the treatment has stopped and the ovaries go back to making testosterone at their previous level. Of course, this is intentional if we want the ovaries to return to normal function in order to get pregnant. It may be therefore that long-term treatment will be required. The usual strategy over time is to use full-dose treatment for between 6 and 24 months to gain maximal effect. Thereafter, the dose is gradually reduced at three to six-monthly intervals to find the lowest dose that maintains the benefit. With any step-down in treatment it is possible that some breakthrough symptoms will emerge and in this way the minimal maintenance level of treatment can be established.

The timing of a pregnancy has to be factored in to the plan for anti-androgen treatment. These drugs have to stop for three months before conceiving as they could have a bad effect on how the fetus develops. The three month gap gives plenty of time for the drugs to leave the system so that the baby can develop in a drug-free environment. This can be a difficult time for women who find that their symptoms bounce back quickly when off treatment. Some advice should be given beforehand about how to shorten the gap between stopping treatment and conceiving. For instance, if periods are known to be very infrequent then it might be an option to proceed to simple fertility treatment such as with clomifene citrate, rather more quickly than usual.

acne

Acne is a common problem in teenagers. When it extends into adult life it can become a part of PCOS. The evidence for this comes from a study of women in a dermatology clinic whose main problem was acne. When an ovary ultrasound was performed, 85% were found to have polycystic ovaries compared to 20% expected as an average for all women.

The cells within the skin that are responsible for making natural skin grease or seborrhoea are sensitive to testosterone. Any condition with a high testosterone level can trigger acne. Similarly, any treatment that lowers the action of testosterone on the skin will improve acne.

The development of a spot on the skin has three phases. Testosterone encourages the sebaceous gland to make more grease than average. The surface of the gland becomes inflamed and a plug made of protein called keratin begins to form over the surface. Once the skin pore has become blocked then an infection with a specific bacterium, *Propionibacterium acnes* sets in.

three phases of acne formation and three different types of treatment

The testosterone-drive to the sebaceous gland can be reduced using all of the treatments described for hirsutism – combined oral contraceptive pills, anti-androgens and metformin. Acne usually responds to these treatments more quickly compared to hirsutism. Therefore, a lower-dose treatment plan can be effective. Studies have shown that acne continues to improve for over nine months when using the combined oral contraceptive. With this fact in mind, it is worth sticking to a treatment plan for some time in order to get really effective results.

The formation of a keratin plug can be prevented using surface retinoids that are similar in structure to vitamin A. These form the basis of many cosmetic acne treatments and act as exfoliants to prevent pores clogging up. Isotretinoin (Accutane or Roaccutane) is a tablet treatment that is only prescribed by dermatology specialists. It can be very effective at suppressing acne and may provide remission for some months or even years. Isotretinion treatment has to be monitored very carefully and has significant side effects including anaemia, hepatitis, depression and inflammation of the eye.

Antibiotics are used to prevent the final phase of acne formation which is the infection of blocked pores by *propionibacterium acnes*. For temporary outbreaks of acne, and in fairly mild situations, antibiotics can work very well and are often the second-line treatment after surface cosmetic treatments. There is always some concern about the effect of long-term antibiotics on the bacteria of the

three stages of acne formation and the action of treatments to block each stage

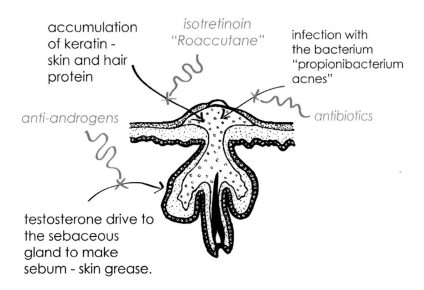

accumulation of keratin - skin and hair protein

isotretinoin "Roaccutane"

infection with the bacterium "propionibacterium acnes"

anti-androgens

antibiotics

testosterone drive to the sebaceous gland to make sebum - skin grease.

bowel and on immunity, but on the whole these treatments are well tolerated. Antibiotics are available either as an application to the skin or as tablets.

Unfortunately there are few trials that compare the side effects and benefits of each treatment approach. Anti-androgens tend to be used by endocrinologists if this is the first point of referral. For women with regular periods who might not be considered as having a significant hormone drive or who may not have the diagnosis of PCOS, the referral pathways are often to dermatology where antibiotics and isotretinion are favoured.

In specialist centres laser treatment is also available for acne but there are few research trials reporting the effectiveness of this form of treatment. Laser might be considered however if there are side effects to the other treatments.

alopecia

Thinning of scalp hair is one of the most distressing symptoms related to PCOS. It can often be the third in the sequence of testosterone-driven symptoms following on from acne and hirsutism. It tends to be the last of these events to appear. Many women troubled by hirsutism, however, will never experience alopecia. In addition, some women may present in the 30s or 40s with alopecia who have never previously experienced acne or hirsutism. In this situation where symptoms of PCOS are not obvious, the diagnosis is never made and anti-androgens are often not offered.

Unlike hirsutism, there are several other factors to consider that might contribute to the risk of scalp hair thinning. First, the genetic predisposition is quite strong and of course this cannot be altered. More important is the impact of other conditions that can make the hair follicles much more fragile. The first of these is an underactive thyroid gland, which should be easily detected as a blood test for thyroid hormones is usually the first test on the list for alopecia.

Second are the vitamins and minerals that support the scalp hair follicle and deficiency of any one of these can cause hair thinning.

The most important deficiency syndrome causing alopecia is that of iron. There might be a past history of iron-deficient anaemia or of very heavy periods which cause excessive iron loss. Most commonly however, iron deficiency is at a low level and only the scalp hair follicle can detect it. There are several blood tests for iron deficiency which include a measurement of iron itself in the circulation, the ability of proteins in the blood to combine with iron – iron binding capacity, and probably most important for its association with hair growth is the measurement of iron stores, *ferritin*. A fact that is often missed is that simply having a ferritin result within the reference range is not sufficient for optimal hair growth. Instead, the aim should be to achieve a serum ferritin in the upper half of the reference range. It can take many months of iron supplements in order to achieve this. Iron is such an important factor for hair growth that it is almost always worth considering a supplement alongside any other treatment. Iron tablets should also contain vitamin C which improves the absorption of iron in the intestine.

Other vitamins and minerals for which the evidence is less clear are still worth checking on a blood test: zinc, vitamin B_{12}, and vitamin D. Once again, even with low normal levels it would be worth considering supplements for zinc and vitamin B complex in order to boost the levels to the upper part of the normal range. The reason for taking this comprehensive approach to treatment is because it can be very difficult to encourage hair follicles on the scalp to start growing again and so pushing every positive factor to the optimal level may be a good investment. Unfortunately, because scalp hair grows so slowly, it is difficult to perform research trials to prove the effectiveness of each of these supplements.

Once all of the issues relating to the thyroid function, vitamins and minerals have been addressed, then anti-androgens can also be considered. Curiously, the blood levels of testosterone are almost always normal when alopecia is a prominent symptom. This must be an indication that it is hair follicle sensitivity that is the main problem rather than testosterone excess. Having said that, reducing exposure to testosterone even when it is in the normal range may well be effective.

All of the treatments described in the section on hirsutism are used in alopecia. Because this symptom often occurs in an older age group, the oral contraceptive may not be suitable and a combination of anti-androgens would be favoured. Most of the evidence from research for treatment with anti-androgens relates to finasteride. Finasteride is favoured because the enzyme that it addresses, 5-alpha reductase, is present in the skin of the scalp. As responses to treatment can be disappointing it is worth considering combining a two-pronged approach using finasteride with spironolactone.

Vitamins and minerals will help to stabilise scalp hair follicles in the resting telogen phase. These supplements together with anti-androgens will work in the growing anagen phase to promote stronger and thicker hair growth. Because of the very long hair-growth cycle on the scalp, it can take many months before the hair density thickens. In addition, scalp hair fall-out can often continue for many weeks even after treatment has started as the current set of hair follicles that are programmed to fall out over subsequent weeks cannot be influenced.

Blood testing is helpful to make sure that any supplement is optimised and that excessive levels have not accumulated in the blood. If spironolactone is used then plasma potassium should be checked every six months with a blood test.

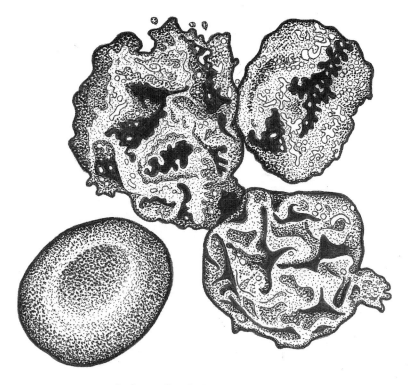

cells from the lining of the womb

The three cells on the right-hand side are skin-like cells or epithelium that form the lining of the womb or endometrium. The round cell at the bottom left is a blood cell that will accompany the epithelial cells in menstrual flow.

chapter 4
irregular periods

what happens to periods in PCOS?

Regular periods occurring every 28 days are a reliable experience for many women. The menstrual cycle however, is a fairly delicate and complex mechanism. There is quite a long list of conditions that will result in a change in the timing of periods or even cause them to stop altogether – *amenorrhoea*. In PCOS, some women may have a completely normal and regular menstrual cycle but it is most common for there to be an unpredictable and prolonged interval between periods which could occur at any time between 5 weeks and 6 months apart – *oligomenorrhoea*. A minority of women with PCOS experience a complete absence of periods for some time in their life.

In PCOS, irregular periods in young life can gradually improve over the years. Paradoxically, some women find that periods become regular only in their 40s. In others, the improvement in periods with age does not occur and so this general rule cannot be relied upon.

A period usually follows two weeks after ovulation. It is unusual to have regular periods but fail to ovulate (although of course this can occur as will be discussed in the chapter on fertility). For many women with irregular periods the main problem with getting pregnant is that one never knows when the fertile time will be as the day of ovulation is so unpredictable.

words used to describe different period patterns

Amenorrhoea – no periods occurring for over six months. There are several conditions that cause periods to stop altogether. When this is the only symptom of PCOS without hirsutism or acne then further testing is required as outlined below.

Dysfunctional uterine bleeding – chaotic unscheduled periods. Periods can be so chaotic that they appear to have no pattern to them and may occur every two weeks. It is not uncommon for there to be a small show of a period at the time of ovulation when there is a slight dip in oestrogen levels. This can give the impression of periods every two weeks but in fact only one of them is a 'real' period. In women with PCOS who have had no period for some time, the surface of the lining of the womb can become unstable and then come away almost non-stop like a period going on for weeks. This is most common in women who are overweight.

Dysmenorrhoea – more than the usual amount of pain during a period. This can be part of PCOS if periods are very delayed and a thick lining means that the flow will also be heavy. Endometriosis is a common cause of dysmenorrhoea when typically there is an onset of severe pain just as the period starts that then wears off slowly until the period stops. Extra painful regular periods are not typical of PCOS and another cause of pain should be sought. Although the ovaries may be larger than average they are very rarely the source of pain.

Menorrhagia – of a period when the flow is heavier than normal. Heaviness of a period is measured both in terms of daily flow rate and length of bleeding time. Heaviness can be hard to quantify but using more than 12 tampons during a period is considered excessive. The average length of a period is five days, and over seven days qualifies for menorrhagia. This can be part of PCOS when the interval since the last period is prolonged. An underactive thyroid gland or being overweight are common causes of menorrhagia.

Oligomenorrhoea – period intervals between 35 days and six months. This is the most typical pattern in PCOS where periods may happen every two to three months. Very few other conditions cause longstanding oligomenorrhoea – most other causes quickly proceed to a complete lack of periods over a few months.

are irregular periods and oligomenorrhoea the same thing?

By using the term irregular periods we usually mean a longer than average interval between periods as in the medical term oligomenorrhoea. Irregular periods can also be used to mean that the heaviness of periods can vary from month to month or that the timing may be off by a few days each month. Traditionally, it is accepted that periods can vary between 25 and 35 days and still be classified as within the normal range. Periods can also be irregular by occurring too frequently, perhaps every two to three weeks. This pattern is not typical of PCOS and therefore would require investigation on its own account.

The average age for starting periods is 13 years old. Periods continue for over 35 years until the menopause occurs around the age of 50. At either end of this age spectrum there are times of irregular periods which are considered to be normal. After periods start it commonly takes one year for the interval between them to settle down into a regular pattern. Therefore it would be unusual to start investigations for periods alone before the age of 14. In a woman's 40s, periods normally come a little closer together and it is not unusual for the period interval to be between 21 and 25 days in the years before the menopause. While the shortened period interval before the menopause is a common experience, almost any pattern and degree of irregular timing can occur, but this seldom causes confusion with PCOS as it would have normally presented earlier in life.

what other reasons are there for the periods to stop and what tests are required?

A textbook would be able to offer a long list of causes of absent periods but only four conditions are common:

- Polycystic ovary syndrome
- Thyroid hormone imbalance
- Raised prolactin
- Early ovarian failure

PCOS is the only one of these common conditions that has features of an excess of testosterone such as hirsutism or acne. Therefore, the presence of these symptoms with irregular periods more or less makes the diagnosis of PCOS – often no further tests are required. PCOS also differs from the other three in that oestrogen levels tend to be normal in PCOS but low in the others. The oestrogen level is best assessed using ultrasound measurement of the endometrium rather than by a blood test. The blood level of oestrogen is very variable depending exactly on the activity of the ovary at the time of the test. The thickness of lining of the womb – the *endometrium* – provides a more reliable measurement that can be considered as a biological measurement of oestrogen levels.

Before ultrasound was available, oestrogen status was tested by giving progesterone for ten days – a *progesterone withdrawal test*. If a period occurred after progesterone then PCOS was a likely cause of amenorrhoea, but if not, one of the other conditions was more likely. This test has largely been abandoned, as it was not very effective compared to ultrasound.

The three other causes of irregular periods can be easily identified with a blood test measuring the following hormones: TSH, thyroxine, prolactin, FSH and LH. In addition, a pelvic ultrasound will also be helpful in most instances.

I have been told that my prolactin is high – what does that mean?

Prolactin is one of the hormones made by the pituitary gland and its main role is in pregnancy to prepare for breast-feeding. Raised prolactin or *hyperprolactinaemia* is a cause of irregular periods as the body thinks that you might be breast-feeding and tries to switch off the ovarian cycle.

Raised prolactin levels can be particularly confusing in relation to PCOS. The reason for this is that a modestly raised prolactin reading, say up to three times the average value, is found in approximately 15% of women with PCOS. Raised prolactin seems to be part of the overall hormone imbalance related to the syndrome. High prolactin levels can also arise from conditions of the pituitary gland such as a prolactin-producing nodule called a prolactinoma. In this situation, the prolactin levels tend to be higher, perhaps ten times the reference level, and the levels of LH, FSH and oestradiol all tend to be lower than in PCOS. Between the two ends of the spectrum is a grey area where it is difficult to work out whether the problem is primarily the pituitary gland or PCOS. Often, it is only after taking several readings over some months that a decision can be made as to which is the most important factor – PCOS or raised prolactin. Sometimes, this situation can be clarified by a trial of treatment. For instance, bromocriptine is one of the standard treatments for raised prolactin and almost always brings the prolactin level into the normal range. If the period pattern becomes normal then this simple treatment can be continued indefinitely. Usually, raised prolactin is a benign self-limiting condition that goes away after three to five years and it only causes inconvenience if it coincides with trying to get pregnant.

how does overweight affect periods?

Women with PCOS who are also overweight are much more likely to have period problems compared to women with PCOS of average bodyweight. Many of the period problems that occur with excess weight will improve with weight loss. There are several mechanisms by which excess weight can affect the period pattern.

First, we have seen in earlier chapters that weight gain causes insulin resistance, and that the high levels of insulin are a drive for the ovary to make more testosterone. Within the ovary, the testosterone slows down the developing follicle causing delayed ovulation. In this way, being overweight causes the polycystic ovary to misbehave more, which is reflected in a longer gap between periods.

Second, fat tissue in the body is an alternative source of oestrogen and the high oestrogen levels encourage further thickening of the endometrium. Fat tissue actively converts male hormones made by the adrenal gland to oestrogen. This extra source of oestrogen causes greater thickening of the endometrium. This mechanism is one of the reasons why women who are overweight are particularly prone to heavy periods. With weight loss this problem resolves.

Lastly, women who have an underactive thyroid gland tend to gain weight because the whole metabolism of the body is running slowly. Thyroid hormone also causes the body to use oestrogen more slowly. As oestrogen lasts longer in the body, so its effect is more pronounced causing a thickened endometrium. This is the reason why women with an underactive thyroid gland often have heavy periods. An underactive thyroid gland occurs more commonly than expected in PCOS and should be looked for particularly in women who have period problems. Periods tend to be lighter again when treatment is started with thyroid hormone supplements – *thyroxine*. It is sometimes surprising that a relatively small degree of underactive thyroid gland can cause quite pronounced period problems. Raised TSH on a thyroid function blood test can easily identify an underactive thyroid gland.

endometrial hyperplasia

One of the most important problems in PCOS is a thickening in the lining of the womb that occurs in women who have infrequent periods. The lining of the womb, or the endometrium, varies between 5 mm just as the period is finishing and then thickens up to about 10 mm at the time of ovulation. If ovulation does not occur then the endometrium can get thicker and thicker, perhaps by as much as 20 mm, if it never receives the signal to come away as a period.

The signal to shed the endometrium to start a period occurs as the levels of progesterone and oestrogen come down at the end of the cycle. It is these two hormones that support the lining. As they fall away it is as if the carpet is pulled away from the structure of the lining and a period occurs. The thicker the lining, the more likely it is that blood clots occur causing the period to be very heavy and painful. If the thickened lining is left indefinitely with a measurement greater than 12 mm, then we apply the term *endometrial hyperplasia*. The word hyperplasia means that the tissue is overgrown. If endometrial hyperplasia is left untreated indefinitely, then there is a risk that it could become cancerous for which the only treatment might be surgical removal of the entire womb – a hysterectomy.

The risk of endometrial hyperplasia has to be taken seriously and it is for this reason that every woman should experience at least four periods per year. For an adequate safety margin however, many gynaecologists will recommend striving for a period every month. Women who are overweight carry the biggest risk of endometrial cancer because of the extra oestrogen drive. Therefore being overweight with oligomenorrhoea always requires treatment.

An ultrasound of the womb is the most effective method of assessing the endometrium. Not only can a measurement be made of the thickness of the lining, but also a judgment can be made as to whether it looks worrying by virtue of having an irregular appearance. A patchiness in the appearance of a thick endometrium means that the condition has been there for some time and needs urgent action. A treatment trial with progesterone is often the first course of action with a repeat ultrasound after an induced period to make sure that the lining thickness has come down. While any of the medical treatments listed below can be effective, the quickest method of receiving reassurance as to whether the lining is a risk for cancer might be to take a biopsy sample.

The endometrium can be examined directly by a simple outpatient procedure called a *hysteroscopy*. This involves inserting a thin optical fibre through the cervix that allows the surface to be seen. Alongside this is a small device that allows biopsy samples to be taken. The samples are then placed on a microscope slide for later analysis. The result of a biopsy of the endometrium usually takes between one and two weeks to come back. If the procedure cannot be carried out in clinic then a more intensive option is to have the examination under anaesthetic with removal of the lining – dilatation and curettage or D&C.

premenstrual symptoms

The hormone progesterone that is made after ovulation causes most of the symptoms that occur in the week before a period. It is sensitivity to progesterone that causes changes in mood, bloatedness and breast tenderness as well as many other symptoms rather than abnormal progesterone levels. Blood tests are therefore not helpful. Progesterone sensitivity can only be assessed by the description of the timing in the cycle. Most women experience these changes to a small degree and for others the premenstrual week can be a devastating experience every month.

Some women who never considered themselves to have premenstrual syndrome, can go through a phase when the symptoms can be very difficult. Occasionally, there is a clear explanation as to why someone enters a phase of progesterone sensitivity. An underactive thyroid gland seems to make premenstrual symptoms worse, and any cause for depression will also bring out PMS even if it is a clear reaction to a life event such as bereavement.

Premenstrual symptoms therefore, are signs that ovulation has occurred and if fertility is the only issue then the symptoms can be a 'good sign'. For instance, for women whose periods become more regular when taking metformin, some will report that overall they feel less well because the premenstrual time is occurring more frequently.

More mysterious are the premenstrual-like symptoms that occur with very delayed periods. These symptoms are very similar to those triggered by progesterone in a regular cycle. Many women with oligomenorrhoea find that they enter a phase of very prolonged premenstrual symptoms that could last for months until a period appears. The symptoms pass as if a cloud is suddenly lifted at the onset of menstruation. The exact hormonal cause of symptoms in this situation is less clear because oligomenorrhoea means that ovulation has not occurred. Therefore it cannot be progesterone that is the source of the problem in oligomenorrhoea. Almost any of the methods described below to address irregular periods will relieve these symptoms although progesterone has to be used cautiously. If someone is sensitive to progesterone in terms of premenstrual symptoms then any treatment containing progesterone can be as bad as the initial problem.

There are other factors apart from progesterone that add to premenstrual symptoms. The uterus makes a variety of inflammation factors or *cytokines* that also cause symptoms. For instance, progesterone-based intrauterine devices (IUD) such as the Mirena device can be very effective at relieving the symptoms of prolonged premenstrual syndrome in oligomenorrhoea. The Mirena does not however, alter the hormone pattern from the ovary. This would suggest that there must be some substance made by the womb that causes havoc in the rest of the body. Progesterone in the uterus appears to dampen down local inflammation.

There are many alternative preparations that are promoted to improve premenstrual symptoms. Given that conventional medical treatment is not always effective in this area, alternative preparations are certainly worth a try. Treatments in this group include vitamin B6, magnesium, tryptophan and evening primrose oil. There are very few scientific trials that are helpful in choosing alternative treatments. This is a particularly difficult area to run scientific trials in because of the overlap between low mood and premenstrual syndrome.

It is thought that serotonin in the brain is one way in which somebody 'detects' progesterone. So the antidepressants family that affect the serotonin system – *selective serotonin re-uptake inhibitors* (or SSRIs) such as fluoxetine (Prozac) – are amongst the most effective of all treatments for premenstrual moods change. Unlike when used for depression, this family of antidepressants can be used for a very low dose for between 10–14 days per month just to cover the premenstrual time and may not need to be used continuously. Although many people are naturally, and quite rightly, wary of antidepressants, used in this way they are certainly worth a try if the mood component to premenstrual syndrome warrants it.

how to control irregular (infrequent) periods

weight loss

As for so many things relating to PCOS, weight loss is top of the agenda for improving problem periods for women who are overweight. Sometimes, weight loss alone can be all that is required and the clue that this may be true is if there is a reference point earlier in life when periods behaved themselves at a lower body weight. Of course, there are many women with PCOS who have irregular periods at an average body weight and so the return of normal periods with weight loss is not guaranteed.

Because weight loss can take some time, it may be that one of the alternatives below will be needed for some months, after which treatment could be stopped so that the natural period interval could be assessed again. Different forms of progesterone and metformin are the mainstay of treatment for women who are overweight and the combined oral contraceptive pills should be avoided because of the extra risk of a blood clot.

combined oral contraceptives

Combined oral contraceptives are often the first form of treatment that doctors turn to in order to control periods. The reason for this is that they have a high success rate and work in almost any situation including PCOS. They are particularly useful if there are symptoms of testosterone excess such as hirsutism or acne. With one treatment, periods can be made regular and the testosterone production from the ovary suppressed at the same time. There is no other treatment that achieves this quite so successfully. Another situation where the pill will always be used first is when this would be a chosen form of contraception.

The downside of the pill is that it is a bit of a crude approach to treatment, bringing about a completely artificial period control and inducing 'fake' periods. This type of treatment certainly would be of no help for a woman who is trying to conceive. There are many groups of women who cannot take the combined pill such as those who are very overweight, smokers or those who suffer migraine headaches. In addition, there are many women who simply do not like the way the pill makes them feel.

There is a commonly held concern that using the pill may in some way have a bad effect on the chances of getting pregnant later in life. There is no scientific evidence that supports this myth so it is often worthwhile considering a course of the pill if only to establish how effective this type of treatment might be as a therapeutic trial. It is perfectly satisfactory to stop the pill at any time – the ovaries will simply return to their previous condition. It is worthwhile however, trying to persist for two to three months to see if any side effects settle before abandoning this treatment altogether. There is no reason why the pill could not be used more or less indefinitely for women who have very irregular periods and who do not have a high risk of a blood clot.

The risks of long-term pill use in PCOS such as a slightly higher risk of breast cancer in women who use the pill for over five or ten years, have to be balanced against the benefits of reducing other forms of cancer such as that of the ovary and particularly endometrial cancer for women with PCOS and oligomenorrhoea. With regard to breast cancer, although it is the pill for which we have the greatest amount of data, there is also concern that long-term use of progesterone might also contribute to breast cancer risk. Therefore, avoiding the pill where there is a small excess risk of breast cancer and replacing it with progesterone for which there is no comparing long-term data for breast cancer may be misguided.

progesterone family

The family of progesterone hormones go under the name of progestogens. There are several forms of progestogen available for use as treatment and there are also different time schedules for using progesterone intermittently to control periods. Progesterone works in two ways to control periods – to trigger shedding of the endometrium when it is already thickened and to prevent endometrial thickening.

Short course – progesterone challenge test or cyclical progesterone treatment. A short 10 to 14-day course of progestogen once per month produces a 'pulse' that mimics the function of the corpus luteum after ovulation. Progestogens supplied as a short course once per month as a cyclical form of treatment is very effective for period control yet without many of the cautions or side effects of the combined oral contraceptive pill. Cyclical progesterone is usually taken between days 16 and 26 of the cycle or for 10 days each month starting randomly for women with irregular periods. One convenient way of remembering this treatment is to take it for the first 10 days of each calendar month. Some doctors favour 12 or 14-day courses each month if periods are difficult to control.

Long course – cyclical progesterone. Progestogens can be used to prevent the build up of the endometrium if given on a longer course each month. In this way, progestogens block the action of oestrogen that thickens up the endometrium. An example of this function is the combined oral contraceptive pills in which progesterone is included in all 21 tablets. In women taking these pills, the lining of the womb rarely thickens to over 5 mm. Progestogens taken on their own for between 21 and 26 days of each cycle will have a similar effect to the combined pill preventing the lining from thickening. The long course of progesterone usually starts three to five days after the period starts. The long course of cyclical progestogen can be effective when the short course does not control periods, but of course it does mean having to take more hormone tablets which may not suit everyone.

four forms of progestogen that are commonly used as cyclical treatment:

Norethisterone in a dose of 5–15 mg per day is the strongest of progestogens. It is the most effective progestogen at ensuring that the lining of the womb is adequately cleared.

Norethisterone is therefore the first treatment that a doctor may choose if the endometrium is markedly thickened. Hand-in-hand with being the most potent progestogen, norethisterone also has the greatest side effects causing some testosterone-like symptoms, particularly acne, and symptoms similar to premenstrual syndrome.

Medroxyprogesterone acetate in a dose of 5–10 mg per day is commonly used to control periods and has rather fewer side effects compared to norethisterone. It is therefore probably the treatment of first choice.

Micronised progesterone (100 to 200 mg) is identical to natural progesterone that is made by the ovary. At first glance this progestogen might be considered to be the best option. In practice, micronised progesterone is the least potent of this group of treatments. Therefore it may not be as effective for long-term control of the endometrium. This treatment however is worth considering as it has the fewest side effects of the progestogen family.

Desogestrel, levonorgestrel and norethindrone are synthetic progestogens that are available in a cyclical calendar pack and marketed as progesterone-only pills (POPs) – eg. Cerazette, Micronor, Norgeston. This treatment can be a very useful option for women who require contraception. POPs may not be as efficient as the other progestogens in controlling periods, particularly if the starting point is a very thickened endometrium. In this situation it might be better to ensure good clearance of the endometrium using medroxyprogesterone acetate for 10 days and then continue thereafter using a POP. This pill is particularly useful for women who are overweight and who therefore cannot take the combined pill because of the risk of thrombosis, and who also require control of oligomenorrhoea.

progestogen inside the uterus

In many ways, it is not logical to bathe the whole body in progestogen when it is only the lining of the womb that requires this hormone in order to prevent excessive thickening. One answer to this conundrum is to use a progestogen that can be inserted into the womb so that only the endometrium sees it.

The Mirena intrauterine device is a form of the coil which contains a pellet of the progestogen *levonorgestrel* that dissolves very gradually over 5 years. This treatment can be very useful for women who find that they are not reliable in taking any form of the pill yet require contraception. The Mirena IUD has the benefit that very little progestogen is absorbed by the body and therefore in theory this should have the fewest side effects of all the progestogen options.

In practice, although this treatment often fulfils its promise, there are some women who are clearly sensitive to even the small amounts of progestogen that are absorbed and then find that the device has to be removed – this is quite a rare event. Of course, the downside of this type of progestogen treatment is the fact that it has to be inserted through the cervix in the same way as any contraceptive coil. *Skyla* has been recently introduced as a slightly lower dose form of levonorgestrel IUD.

metformin

The use of metformin for period control is often under-estimated. Although metformin is not as fool-proof as the combined oral contraceptive or progestogens, it does have its place for some women with PCOS. A proportion of women who take metformin find that the interval between periods get shorter and can approach a normal 28-day cycle. It may be fewer than half of women who take metformin who experience this benefit but for those who do, it provides a useful option.

the use of progesterone to control periods

Examples of two progesterone regimes for controlling the thickness of the lining of the womb. The long course from days 5 - 26 prevents the lining from building up. The short course mimics the natural progesterone surge and triggers shedding of the thickened lining. Each will be used in different situations. It is the short course that is most commonly used.

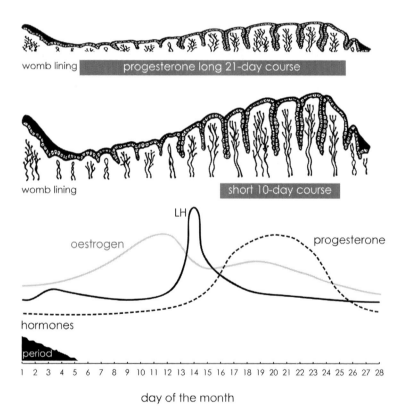

womb lining | progesterone long 21-day course

womb lining | short 10-day course

LH

oestrogen

progesterone

hormones

period

1 2 3 4 5 6 7 8 9 10 11 12 13 14 15 16 17 18 19 20 21 22 23 24 25 26 27 28

day of the month

The situation where metformin might be particularly useful is for a woman who is preparing to get pregnant in the near future. If pregnancy is planned but not an urgency then it would be worth a trial of metformin for at least 6 months to see if a regular menstrual cycle emerges. Even if a pregnancy is not planned, metformin may be useful in women who are overweight who wish to test whether a natural ovulatory cycle can be achieved as opposed to the fake periods that are brought about by the pill or progestogens. If metformin works efficiently then it may also be favoured because the hormone pattern from the ovary is more natural as opposed to taking hormones by tablet.

For women with very irregular periods who find that metformin has had no significant benefit after 6 months, it is probably worth changing on to one of the hormone-based treatments outlined above, particularly if periods are so infrequent as to make endometrial hyperplasia a risk.

As metformin is not as efficient as the hormone-based treatments, and if the lining of the womb is found to be markedly thickened, say over 12 mm, then it is prudent to clear the endometrium with a short course of medroxyprogesterone acetate at the start of metformin treatment whilst waiting for the effect of metformin to build over the following months. It must be remembered that metformin can take some months to work and so this form of treatment cannot be used to urgently address a thickened endometrium.

clomifene citrate

In the past, clomifene has been used on a regular basis to stimulate ovulation and thereby provide regular periods. Because there is no safety data about the long-term use of clomifene, this option is no longer recommended. Clomifene should only be used as a short-term fertility treatment.

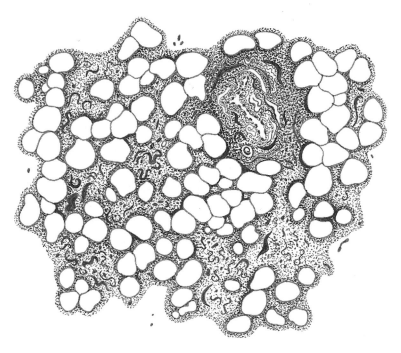

fat cells

This is a diagram of a collection of fat cells that are shown as clear because they are full of fat droplets. The squiggly lines are blood vessels and the irregular shape near the top right is a larger blood vessel. Fat cells are called adipocytes and this diagram represents a sample of adipose tissue.

chapter 5

weight gain and insulin resistance

Excess weight will have different effects on each individual. Some women will be very overweight yet have regular periods with clear skin and therefore no sign of PCOS. Others will only have to gain a few pounds before signs of PCOS appear – often, it is irregular periods or acne that are the first to become evident with weight gain. Symptoms that come on with weight gain are an important clue as to how much improvement might be achieved with weight loss. For instance, if there is a reference point in the past when at a lower body weight there were few signs of PCOS, then one can hope that by returning to this weight, any new symptoms will gradually resolve. In some women, symptoms of PCOS almost disappear with weight loss. Of course, if there is no clear reference point in the past then it may be difficult to predict the extent to which weight loss will be effective. It is as if the ovaries are very sensitive to weight change in some people but not others.

how important is body shape?

One of the ways in which individuals differ is in how they carry their weight – often referred to as apple or pear distribution. The apple shape refers to fat tissue collecting around the waist, while for the pear shape weight is mainly on the thighs. In medical terms, weight gain in the apple variety is of a *central distribution* with more fat tissue surrounding the internal organs of the abdomen. The pear has a *lower segment* weight distribution. The two types of weight distribution also differ in their metabolism and in particular their levels of insulin in circulation.

With the apple distribution the body is more resistant to the action of insulin so the circulating concentrations of insulin are higher compared to the pear distribution. That is, the apple type is more insulin resistant and the pear is more insulin sensitive. The ovary responds to the insulin level and so will misbehave more in women with the apple distribution, whilst the ovaries in someone with the pear distribution will not be so affected by weight change.

how does insulin resistance come about?

The main function of insulin is to control the balance of glucose in the body. When the basic sugar glucose arrives in the blood after eating, the pancreas is activated to make insulin. Insulin in turn allows glucose to pass into cells either for the storage of energy as in fat cells, or for using energy as in muscles. In some instances, insulin can be very efficient in controlling glucose so that only a low level circulates in the blood. In other circumstances insulin can become inefficient and high levels are required to keep the blood glucose normal. When the insulin system is not efficient the term *insulin resistance* is used. Eventually, if glucose cannot be kept within the normal range no matter how high the insulin level, then the level of glucose rises – this is type 2 diabetes. In this way, insulin resistance is a forerunner of diabetes.

One reason why the insulin system may become less efficient is because of weight gain – more and more insulin is required to service an increased amount of fat tissue. A second reason is through genetic programming. Whether one has a genetic tendency to insulin resistance can be estimated by how many relatives there are with type 2 diabetes. Insulin resistance is very strongly inherited. Of course, an overweight person with two parents who have type 2 diabetes is extremely likely to have insulin resistance and to go on to develop diabetes themselves.

Insulin resistance is technically very difficult to measure accurately on blood testing. An estimate can be achieved by measuring the relationship between fasting glucose and fasting insulin measurements or by measuring compounds in the blood that are sensitive to insulin resistance such as SHBG or HDL cholesterol.

The main organs in the body that use a lot of glucose are the liver and the muscles. These organs therefore set the pace for the level of insulin in the body. If either of these two tissues require more glucose, then the level of insulin will rise leading to insulin resistance.

The ovary remains sensitive to insulin even when the rest of the body has become resistant. In this way, when the blood level of insulin is low (an insulin <u>sensitive</u> person), then very little drive is picked up by the ovary. Conversely, in someone who is very insulin resistant in whom the level of insulin is high, the ovary begins to pick up the signal of insulin and responds by producing more testosterone.

how much of my weight problem did I get from my parents?

Being overweight can run in families although sometimes it is not obvious where the problem comes from. Daughters tend to follow the weight trend of their mother and father. Some of this familial tendency can be from genes (nature) and some can be from family habits (nurture). There are many things that we get from parents apart from just the

how insulin resistance works

INSULIN SENSITIVE: In the insulin <u>sensitive</u> state only a small amount of insulin is made by the pancreas to drive the target tissues of liver, muscle and fat cells - the ovary sees very little of it.

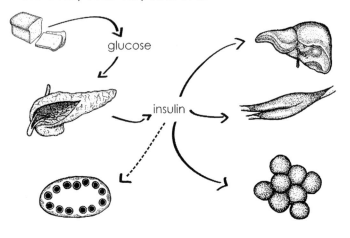

INSULIN RESISTANCE: In the insulin <u>resistant</u> state the circulating level of insulin has to be higher to drive the target tissues and the ovary picks up a significant drive from this to make testosterone.

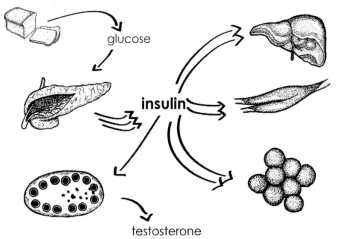

genes that formed us! For one thing, we take on the eating habits of our family. Parents who eat healthy natural food with set meal times pass on good eating habits to their children. Similarly, if you grow up in a family in which regular exercise is commonplace then being fit becomes a natural part of life instead of a battle. The lifestyle of your family is not set in stone however. If during childhood the family setting was one with a lot of junk food and little exercise then these bad habits can be slowly changed but it does take time. Your genes however cannot be changed!

In scientific research, one of the ways in which the impact of genes is investigated is by seeing how twins behave. There are some sets of twins who are separated early in life. They therefore have different experience of lifestyles. By looking at the weight change many years later, it can be calculated how much the genes contributed to weight gain – how much was nature instead of nurture.

It turns out that twins who were raised apart have a very similar body weight to each other, to the same extent as twins who were raised together. This is one of the key pieces of evidence that led to the search for genes that control the accumulation of fat tissue.

Several genes are known to affect body weight. The FTO gene is one example of a single change in one's DNA that can determine how likely you are to be overweight. FTO stands for *fat mass and obesity associated protein*. In an overweight population, a greater than expected proportion will carry this genetic change. The FTO gene has been shown to be associated with type 2 diabetes and polycystic ovary syndrome. In PCOS the effect of the FTO gene seems to be greater than that for the general population. This is an interesting piece of research but there is no way of having a test for FTO in routine practice.

is it my metabolism that makes it hard to lose weight?

The body weight of a person is determined by the balance between the amount of calories being burned and the amount of calories consumed in the diet. The amount of calories being burned is made up of those that are part of the body's settings in the resting state (the *basal metabolic rate* or BMR – not to be confused with body mass index or BMI) and the calories burned up in taking extra exercise. For most people it is the BMR that accounts for the larger amount of energy burning.

Basal metabolic rate is the amount of energy that we use up just breathing, eating and moving about each day – not

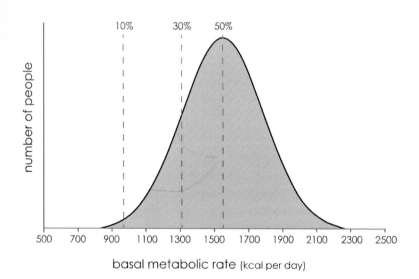

distribution of basal metabolic rates for a 70 kg woman aged 25

BMR is partly programmed by genes. BMR for the average for women is 1550 kcal per day labeled as 50% on the graph above. For one third of women the BMR is 1310 kcal per day labeled as 30%. For an unlucky 10%, it is only 975 kcal per day.

including the amount of energy used up in exercise. One way in which our genes may set our ability to lose weight is by determining our BMR. The average BMR for women is 1500 kcals per day and for men 1700 kcals. This extra burning power in men is the reason why men lose weight more easily than women on the whole. For women, 1500 kcals per day is an average and of course there is great individual variation from about 1100 to 1800 calories per day. So the person with the lowest BMR would have to run about 10 kilometers per day to keep her weight steady if she ate the same as the person with the highest BMR. Exercise has an immediate effect on raising the metabolic rate but only a small lasting effect on the metabolic rate for the rest of the day.

Measuring BMR in the laboratory is not simple. The measurement is made over several hours by putting someone in a controlled space and measuring the heat given off or the amount of carbon dioxide breathed out.

There are various ways of estimating your own BMR based on your age, height, weight and activity level and these can be found on the Internet. These equations give you the average but not your own personal setting. Also, learning this number and balancing it against the calorie content of food intake is not likely to be a productive route to weight loss. It is much better to find a practical way to weight control by your own experience.

One depressing fact of life is that the BMR falls with age. This means it gets harder to lose weight with each passing year. As a consequence everyone needs to be more careful with exercise and diet as they grow older.

the components of food

Everything that we eat can be categorised into five categories: proteins, fats, carbohydrates, fibre and vitamins and minerals.

Protein – this comes from meat, fish, dairy products and pulses. Proteins are important as the body uses them to maintain muscle. Some proteins such as red meats come with unavoidable fat which is why chicken and fish is often favoured. Pulses are a good source of protein as they come with complex slow-release carbohydrate and little fat.

Fat – mostly this is obvious as parts of meat, full-fat dairy and oils used in fried food. All fat has the same high calorie content but some are better for you than others, depending on their effect on cholesterol and heart disease. Fish oils and olive oils are the best for heart disease risk but still have the same amount of calories as the bad forms of animal fat.

Carbohydrate – this group includes bread, potatoes, rice and pasta. Carbohydrates are made up of long chains of sugars and are broken down for processing by the body. The most refined form of carbohydrate are sugars themselves. All sugars are bad for you, although we can accept some that occur naturally in fruit. It is said that 100 years ago we ate an average of 500 g of refined sugar per year and now it is over 500 g per week! Sugar is a potent stimulus to the pancreas to make insulin which, as we have learned, is picked up by the ovary.

The next most refined group of carbohydrates are all white foods – bread, rice and pasta. These have had most of the fibre removed from them and so are absorbed more quickly than brown, less processed forms of food. White bread is turned into sugar more quickly than brown bread. Foods that are high in fibre help to retain some sugars in the intestines which delays their absorption so that the body can use them more efficiently. As a result less insulin is made. The fibre from pulses such as beans and lentils are an example of this effect.

Fibre – this is a good component in food, binding glucose in the intestine so that it is released slowly for absorption. Fibre types such as cellulose and lignin also act as bulking agents which help stave off hunger – these are available in vegetables. Fibre is in fact a form of complex carbohydrate that is not easily broken down. Humans lack the enzyme required to digest cellulose – unlike cows! The only disadvantage from fibre in food is the tendency to cause gas production, resulting in flatulence and bloating. For each individual it may be possible to identify specific forms of fibre that do not have these side-effects and which can then be used freely. For instance, wheat-based fibre commonly causes more side effects than other forms.

Vitamins and minerals – with a healthy diet of natural food, it is rare that vitamin supplements are required. The two that sometimes come up in relation to PCOS are iron and vitamin B_{12}. Iron measured as ferritin in the blood, can run low in those with heavy periods. Low ferritin is associated with scalp hair thinning or alopecia. The absorption of vitamin B_{12} can be impaired by treatment with metformin. People who use metformin for over six months should have a vitamin B_{12} measurement taken once per year.

the problem with processed food

Fast foods are appealing <u>because</u> they contain things that are bad for you. Intense flavours such as sugar and salt make fast foods sell well while fat and refined carbohydrates are cheap fillers. As a general principle anything prepared in a factory or even wrapped in plastic is worth avoiding. Natural raw food is a better alternative.

what is the glycaemic index?

The *glycaemic index* (GI) of foods is a measure of how quickly each type of food appears as sugar in the blood stream after it is absorbed from the intestine. Foods that have a high glycaemic index are absorbed quickly as sugar resulting in a sharp rise in insulin. Pure sugar has the highest glycaemic index. Low glycaemic index foods are absorbed and converted to sugar slowly. Low GI foods are generally the best type for women with PCOS. This principle is the basis of the low-GI diet. List of the GI rating for all types of food are found on the Internet.

is it my ovaries that make me overweight?

Because many women with PCOS have such a battle with weight control, it is often presumed that it is the ovaries that are the cause of the problem. In fact there is little evidence in medicine to support this. In the rare circumstances when ovaries are removed from women with PCOS who are overweight, the metabolism does not seem to change so weight loss is not guaranteed even in this case.

The most likely scenario is that being overweight and PCOS are inherited separately. It is when the two occur together that problems arise. Women who have either polycystic ovaries or weight gain are less likely to come to clinic than those who have both together. For the most part, it is the excess weight that causes otherwise quiet polycystic ovaries to misbehave rather than it being the ovaries which are causing the weight gain.

There is however, an interesting observation suggesting that the polycystic ovary might have a greater effect on weight control than the medical community usually accepts. Some women with PCOS start taking the combined oral contraceptive pill quite early in their teenage life but then find that weight gain only begins to show itself when the pill is stopped maybe 10 or 15 years later. Quite what is happening here is uncertain. This scenario suggests that it is when the ovary wakes up that the metabolism begins to cause problems. Perhaps it is the result of the hormone imbalance from the ovary after all? There has been very little research focusing on this topic and so a scientific explanation is lacking.

what is the best diet for me?

There have been many fads for the perfect diet, some of which make more sense than others! Most sensible diets work on the basic instruction of limiting fat to a minimum and keeping the portions of carbohydrate small with as little refined food as possible. If you are trying to limit both fat and carbohydrate then what is left? Lean protein is still on the menu together with green vegetables and salad, and these should be found in each meal as they provide the bulk that might have come from starch food. Also, beans and lentils – the pulses – should have a prominent place in each day. Diets are covered in more detail in chapter 9.

what about very low-calorie diets?

It is tempting to severely cut the calories to less than 1000 kcals per day or to use liquid replacement diets. The problem with these diets is that they are short-lived and as soon as normal eating is resumed, the weight bounces straight back. It is a rare person who can use this type of diet to start weight loss and then maintain a lower weight or continue to lose weight more slowly with normal food. Also the first 4 kg of weight loss with severe diet restriction is water loss and this is taken back on board as soon as the diet stops. This is why so many diets 'guarantee' weight loss in the first two weeks but they forget to tell you about what follows!

In a way, very low-calorie diets are missing the point. For the long term, the aim is to achieve a new eating behaviour and a sustainable way of living with a weight that one is happy with. Some women describe the problem as a battle between the part of the brain that tempts us to eat the wrong type of food and the part that knows what the body really needs. The core issue is how we deal with the unfairness of the battle – especially when there are people around us who do not seem to need the same restriction. This is why the help of a psychologist can be very successful for weight control. There are simple tools that reinforce our determination to set positive realistic goals and then succeed in achieving them.

There are some exceptional circumstances when a severe diet might be considered such as when there is a short time before trying to get pregnant or to help make a fertility treatment work better at a lower body weight. Even so, a careful plan would need to be in place of how to stop the bounce-back.

surgery for weight loss

While in theory it should always be possible to eat less than the body burns to lose weight, in real life the battle can be almost impossible to win. Operations for weight loss come under the heading of *bariatric surgery* and include gastric band and stomach bypass. These operations came into wider use when the keyhole procedure made them much safer than earlier open surgery.

Bariatric surgery has been shown to be very effective for women with PCOS. For some overweight women with PCOS, many of the symptoms can almost disappear after surgery. One time when such an extreme measure might be considered is when a very overweight woman in her mid-thirties requires fertility treatment because of failure to ovulate. For this group of women, time is of the essence as the supply of eggs is getting smaller but it may take many months before the weight comes down by diet and exercise alone. Having said this, most surgery teams advise that pregnancy is not attempted for 18 months after the operation when the weight loss has stopped. This is because there can be times during rapid weight loss when vitamins and minerals are running low or when protein loss is a problem. Also, it is important to know that a healthy constant weight is stable so as not to cause problems for the nutrient supply for the baby. On the whole, it seems fine to have a pregnancy after bariatric surgery.

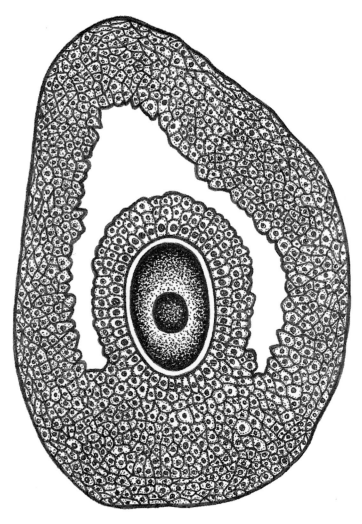

Graafian follicle

This diagram of a follicle within the ovary shows the egg or oocyte at the centre surrounded by granulosa cells. Granulosa cells convert testosterone to oestrogen. The clear area in the middle of the follicle is filled with follicular fluid. The name Graafian comes from Reinier de Graaf (1641–1673). He was a Dutch specialist in anatomy who wrote several works in biology around 1672.

chapter 6
ovulation and fertility

introduction

Many women with PCOS will get pregnant without delay. This may be surprising for someone in whom PCOS was only discovered because of difficulty conceiving. In general you can tell how easy it will be to get pregnant by how regular the menstrual cycle is. For instance, women for whom the main problem is hirsutism are likely to be normally fertile if they have a regular menstrual cycle. Even if the periods are up to 60 days apart, many women will conceive over some months. Fertility treatment will be required, however, when the cycle is prolonged – with more than 2 months between periods. It is all to do with how often an egg is released; ovulation is everything.

Taking all of the treatment options into account, for women with PCOS who can achieve normal body weight and are below the age of 38, the overall chance of getting pregnant is normal – around 90%. Apart from ovulation status, the most important factor affecting the ability to get pregnant is age (no, it's not body weight this time – although that is the second most important). After the age of 38 all success rates are reduced in all women.

For a woman who has a regular 28-day cycle, the average day for releasing an egg, and the time when she is most fertile, is day 14 of the cycle – exactly halfway between the start of each period. If periods become delayed, then it is the first half of the cycle that is variable. Ovulation still happens two weeks before the period. For instance, a woman who has a regular 35-day cycle will ovulate on approximately day 21.

Everything is relatively simple if the timing between periods is predictable. The difficulty comes when one cycle is 28 days long and then the next one is 40 days long. Ovulation in these two cycles would occur therefore on day 14 and day 26 and so the problem is in knowing when the fertile time will be. It is said that if a couple have intercourse twice per week then it is likely that every ovulation will be adequately covered. On the other hand, it is easy to miss an ovulation if you simply do not know when it will occur. Because of this problem, there are several ways of pinpointing the timing of ovulation as discussed below.

As always, there are exceptions to every rule. Although rare, some women with a perfectly regular menstrual cycle can fail to ovulate. Equally, women who have only one or two periods per year may get pregnant without our assistance if intercourse happens to coincide with a random ovulation.

In up to 20% of infertile couples, all fertility tests turn out to be normal – ovulation occurs every month, the sperm count is normal and the fallopian tubes are completely clear. In this situation, the slightly unhelpful label of *unexplained infertility* is applied which is simply a way of saying that we have no idea why pregnancy is not happening.

how do I know if I ovulate?

Many women can feel when they ovulate. As the dominant follicle bursts on the surface of the ovary it produces a characteristic discomfort. While this symptom can be very reliable for some women, others will have to resort to other methods to know when they ovulate. If ovulation is happening reliably, then PCOS is not likely to be the cause of infertility and tests should focus elsewhere.

testing for ovulation

Three tests for ovulation. The temperature rise does not work well for everyone. Ovulation testing kits detect LH in the urine. The day 21 progesterone test is a blood sample that is sent off to the laboratory. For most purposes the home ovulation kits do the job. The most fertile time is the 48 hours after the test shows positive.

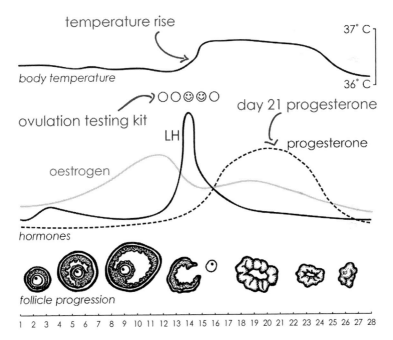

temperature rise

37° C

body temperature

36° C

○○☺☺○   day 21 progesterone

ovulation testing kit

LH

progesterone

oestrogen

hormones

follicle progression

1 2 3 4 5 6 7 8 9 10 11 12 13 14 15 16 17 18 19 20 21 22 23 24 25 26 27 28

day of the month

Finding out when ovulation occurs can be particularly important for women with PCOS who have an unpredictable interval between periods. Often, the only delay in conceiving is finding out when the fertile time is – so that you know when intercourse is likely to be successful.

physical signs of ovulation

There are several signs in the body that ovulation has occurred. These are mainly the result of changes brought about by progesterone which is made only after ovulation. Progesterone causes a slight rise in body temperature of between 0.5 and 1.0°C. By carefully measuring the body temperature every morning it is possible to detect the day of ovulation. While this method has been relied upon in history, it does not work very well for all women, as it is not precise enough to be helpful. In some women the rise in body temperature is just not clear-cut.

A second physical sign that is even more difficult to use is the thinning of mucus coming from the cervix that occurs just after ovulation.

home ovulation testing kits

Home testing kits are designed to detect the hormone luteinizing hormone (LH) in the urine. LH in the blood reaches a sharp peak just before ovulation when some of this hormone also appears in the urine. Usually five dipsticks are provided in each pack to use once per day for five days. On a 28-day cycle it is usual to start checking on day 12 so that you might have two negative results and then a positive on day 14 and 15. An alternative digital system is designed to monitor both LH and oestrogen throughout the cycle with an electronic kit, marketed both as a form of natural contraception (by avoiding the time of ovulation) and as a predictor of ovulation.

In PCOS, there are two problems with LH detector kits. First, the kits are quite expensive. If you are using only one pack per month then the cost may be acceptable. For a woman with an unpredictable cycle however, checking may start on day 12 but ovulation may not happen until day 25 – three kits later! More importantly, the kits simply cannot be used for women who naturally run a high LH measurement as part of the picture of PCOS. The hormone LH is raised in approximately 30% of women with PCOS. This is enough to show as possible ovulation with the kits. You should be suspicious of this if you get continuous weak positive results. To enable the kits to be used in an effective way, it is always advisable to have a measurement of LH taken in the first week after the start of a period. This will establish the LH level that is usually similar in each cycle.

day 21 progesterone

As part of the workup for fertility a doctor may order a measurement of progesterone to be taken approximately one week after ovulation. The peak of progesterone that occurs at this time is a good laboratory method of confirming that ovulation has taken place. This test is often called *Day 21 progesterone* because it is normally on the twenty-first day in a 28-day cycle that progesterone reaches its peak. Any value greater than 25 nmol/L indicates ovulation. For comparison, before ovulation the progesterone measurement in the blood is less than 2 nmol/L. Once again, this test is only reliable if the menstrual cycle is regular. The progesterone result can only be interpreted if we know that the test was taken one week before a period. A low value on this test often simply means that the sample was taken at the wrong time.

ovulation tracking by ultrasound

The Rolls-Royce method of checking ovulation is by using ultrasound scans every few days to watch the ovary as *polycystic ovary syndrome*

an example of a worksheet recording ovulation tracking by ultrasound

Fertility Clinic

Name:
Diagnosis:
Cycle Number:

Day	1	2	3	4	5	6	7	8	9	10	11	12	13	14	15	16	17	18	19	20	21	22	23	24	25	26	27	28	29	30
Date	18	19	20	21	22	23	24	25	26	27	28	29	30	1	2	3	4	5	6	7	8	9	10	11	12	13	14	15	16	17
FSH	4.2																													
LH	9.6											29	21																	
E2	168												1490									90								
Prog																														

monitoring the hormones

Follicles

a follicle ready to ovulate

the corpus luteum

small follicles that don't progress

	1	2	3	4	5	6	7	8	9	10	11	12	13	14	15	16	17	18	19	20	21	22	23	24	25	26	27	28	29	30
24																														
23																														
22																														
21																														
20																														
19																														
18																														
17																														
16																														
15																														
14																														
13																														
12																														
11																														
10																														
9																														
6 – 8																														
≤5																														

monitoring the womb lining

Endo	5						7		9		10														12 Bright					
Drug																														
Dose																														

follicles develop. Once the follicles reach a measurement greater than 10 mm they progress quite reliably, growing at 2 mm per day and then proceed to ovulation when they measure 20 mm. Ultrasound has the benefit over all others methods by being able to predict a few days ahead of time when ovulation will occur. It is helpful to combine this test with a home ovulation testing kit and perhaps also with a day 21 progesterone so that agreement can be achieved using the three methods. In this way the utility of home testing can be established with confidence. The system of ultrasound tracking is just the same as that used to monitor fertility treatments.

After ovulation there is a characteristic appearance of the ovary when the corpus luteum becomes visible and the endometrium takes on a triple line appearance instead of two lines that are seen earlier in the cycle. This means that the lining is prepared for implantation of the embryo.

often there is more than one reason for a couple to be infertile

Infertility is common and is said to affect one in 10 couples. It is usually defined as when a couple have failed to conceive after one year of trying, but many couples will seek advice after six months or even earlier if periods are completely absent. If periods are very infrequent then it seems logical to assume that a failure to ovulate is the cause for infertility. Often there is more than one reason for a couple to be infertile. Before embarking on any treatment therefore, it is important to have a full fertility work-up.

low sperm count

Men can produce anything up to 200 million sperm in each ejaculate. The lower limit of normal is 15 million per millilitre. Low sperm count for men is an increasingly common problem. It is important that a semen analysis is performed early in the process of fertility assessment. There is simply no point of starting treatment for a woman to ovulate only to find that the sperm count is too low for pregnancy to occur. A general practitioner can order a semen analysis but this might have to be repeated in a specialist fertility laboratory if a low count is found. One reason for the repeat test is that the number of sperm can vary from one month to the next. Also, specialist fertility laboratories will undertake more detailed tests of sperm function in order to help work out what level of treatment might be required for the couple.

A semen analysis report will produce a series of numbers relating to the number of sperm as well as the shape and swimming power (mobility) of the sperm. The two most important numbers are the sperm concentration and the sperm mobility – often also called sperm progression. A sperm concentration greater than 15 million per millilitre is considered normal. If the count is between 5 and 15 million a fertility clinic may advise boosting the effect of sperm by using *intra-uterine insemination* (IUI). In this procedure, the good sperm are concentrated and then inserted straight into the womb through the cervix so that they are placed nearer the egg which is coming down the fallopian tube. IUI has been shown to improve fertility outcome for couples with a modestly low sperm count.

With a sperm count below 5 million, it may be that the couple would do better proceeding straight to in-vitro fertilisation (IVF) which makes available an add-on procedure called *intra-cytoplasmic sperm injection* (ICSI) – pronounced icksee. This procedure involves injecting a single sperm directly into the egg that is held on the end of a glass pipette by slight suction. This is a specialist procedure that is only available in IVF clinics.

blocked fallopian tubes

If it has been established that the male contribution to fertility is satisfactory, then the last factor to check is whether there is a clear passage for the sperm and egg to meet. The most vulnerable area for an obstruction is the *fallopian tube* that connects the uterus to the ovaries. Fallopian tubes can become blocked by infections such as chlamydia or by endometriosis. The fallopian tubes can be checked by several procedures:

HyCoSy – (Hysterosalpingo-Contrast-Sonography): ultrasound assessment of the uterus and tubes using a special contrast media

Hysterosalpingogram – an x-ray procedure with dye inserted through the cervix

Lap and Dye – a laparoscope is passed through the tummy button so that the ends of the tubes can be seen by direct vision. The tubes are checked with dye inserted through the cervix under general anaesthetic.

Whilst there are procedures to try to unblock fallopian tubes, most couples are advised to proceed straight to IVF if the tubes are blocked. During IVF the fallopian tube is bypassed completely as the eggs are moved from the ovary and the fertilised embryo is placed into the womb.

low ovarian reserve

As the number of eggs within the ovaries decline with the years, so the chances of getting pregnant are reduced. The chances of ovulation and fertilisation are less with a lower number of eggs. There are various ways of estimating how many eggs are left. The age of a woman is probably the most important factor. Over the age of 38 there is a noticeably lower chance of getting pregnant. A raised concentration of FSH or a low level of AMH are also signs of few eggs remaining or low ovarian reserve. On ultrasound the number of small antral follicles is an indicator of total egg numbers – expressed as an *antral follicle count* or AFC. FSH, AMH and AFC are usually measured before every IVF cycle. For a routine fertility workup FSH alone is usually sufficient.

treatments to make ovulation happen

weight loss

While some women who are very overweight seem to have no trouble getting pregnant, it is also true that being overweight is a major problem causing infertility in women with PCOS. Therefore, once again, weight loss is top of the list of important points for an overweight woman who is trying to conceive.

The main reason for emphasising weight is that all fertility treatments are more effective at a lower body weight. Indeed, there are many fertility centres who will not treat women who are overweight simply because the success rate is so low. In the NHS, fertility treatment is not usually offered if the BMI is over 30 kg/m^2.

Some women with PCOS may be normally fertile at a lower body weight and it is only the weight gain that is driving the failure of ovulation. Women with infrequent periods who can think back to a time when they were at a lower body weight and had regular periods are of a group for whom weight loss may be the only treatment required. It is also possible to have infrequent periods at a normal body weight so not everyone will succeed by weight loss alone.

Another reason why weight loss is so important is for the health of a pregnancy. Overweight women with PCOS are at a higher risk of having diabetes in pregnancy. This risk can be reduced if time is taken to lose weight before conceiving. Excess weight not only puts a hold on ovulation but also increases the risk of miscarriage. In fact, it is the only risk factor for miscarriage that can be reduced by lifestyle measures alone.

There is no absolute cut-off in weight that has to be achieved to make fertility better. While a strict goal would be to achieve a body mass index of 25 kg/m^2, anything below 30 kg/m^2 is likely to be OK.

fertility treatments – ovulation induction

Fertility treatments for women with PCOS who do not ovulate are designed to stimulate the ovaries to release a single egg – *ovulation induction*. The aim of ovulation induction is to produce an ovulation with a single dominant follicle. With treatment, however, more than one follicle can be produced and so the risk of having twins is increased from a background risk of one in 80, to a risk of approximately one in 10. The risk of having twins can be reduced with careful monitoring by ultrasound. If several mature follicles are identified then pregnancy should be avoided for that month. For this reason monitoring by ultrasound should be part of all attempts at ovulation induction . There are two types of ovulation induction – tablets and injections.

clomifene citrate – clomid

Since the early 1960s Clomifene citrate has been the mainstay of fertility treatment for women with PCOS who fail to ovulate. Clomifene works by being an *anti-oestrogen*. Oestrogen in the circulation has a negative feedback on the pituitary to hold down the output of LH and FSH. An anti-oestrogen will release the pituitary from this braking system and results in higher levels of LH and FSH. These two hormones then pass through the blood stream to the ovary where they stimulate the growth of the follicle and the release of the egg.

Clomifene has a high success rate with approximately 75% of women ovulating after taking this treatment. After three treatment cycles over 50% of women will get pregnant.

Clomifene is taken for only five days at the beginning of the menstrual cycle. Counting the first day of the period as day one, clomifene is usually taken between days two and six inclusively. An alternative regime uses clomifene between days five and nine and there is no obvious difference between these two strategies.

The starting dose of clomifene is 50 mg per day increasing each month to 100 mg for five days and then to 150 mg for five days – a higher dose is necessary only if ovulation does not occur at the lower dose. For women who have more than one follicle develop with clomifene 50 mg, the dose can be reduced the next month to 25 mg for five days.

In earlier times, clomifene was prescribed without any ultrasound monitoring. It was a bit of pot luck whether the treatment worked as no one had any idea when or if ovulation might occur. More seriously, some women had a very sprightly response to clomifene producing several eggs at once resulting in a risk of twins or triplets or even more babies. The reports that you may remember of women having five or six babies usually came from clomifene treatment in the days before monitoring was used.

Ultrasound monitoring of clomifene usually starts two to four days after the last period so that the maturing follicle can be tracked and the day of ovulation estimated. Subsequent scans are arranged depending on how the follicle is growing. In this way the best timing of intercourse can be identified. Monitoring in this way has the additional benefit that the success of ovulation can be seen right away so that if ovulation fails to occur then the dose can be altered or a different level of treatment can be chosen for the next cycle. In many centres, once the first cycle of Clomid is complete and if ovulation looks straightforward, then a second cycle might go ahead with only home ovulation kit testing but without ultrasound monitoring. If several follicles are seen that are all of a size that might ovulate then the cycle should be abandoned. Intercourse is avoided or barrier contraception used.

Sometimes, additional treatments are added to a treatment cycle with clomifene but in fact they are rarely needed. Ovulation can be triggered with the hormone *human chorionic gonadotrophin* (hCG) but research studies have shown that ovulation should occur naturally so hCG is of no benefit. After ovulation there is sometimes a recommendation to add progesterone in order to boost the progesterone that should be coming from the corpus luteum. This form of treatment goes under the name of *luteal phase support*. While this treatment is required in IVF, it is of no benefit with treatment using clomifene.

If ovulation does not occur with clomifene then this treatment is not worth pursuing and a more effective alternative is required. Of course, just because ovulation can be made to happen, does not mean that a pregnancy is guaranteed. If pregnancy does not happen after several successful ovulations then a review of other causes of infertility should be made.

Before starting this type of fertility treatment, the male side will have been checked with a sperm count. If there is any question that the sperm count is below average then the addition of intra-uterine insemination can be added to treatment with clomifene citrate.

alternatives to clomifene

There are two other types of anti-oestrogen that have been used but there is relatively little information about their use. Tamoxifen is very similar to clomid in its actions and has no proven benefit.

Letrozole is an alternative that works in a slightly different way to clomifene but it has the same effect of increasing the FSH drive to the ovary. Letrozole blocks the conversion of testosterone to oestrogen resulting in a fall in oestrogen levels and a then a boost of LH and FSH. The largest trial of Letrozole shows that it is more effective than clomid with a higher live birth rate. The improved results with Letrozole were particularly obvious in women who were overweight (BMI greater than 30 kg/m^2). There was no benefit for women with a BMI less than 30 kg/m^2. Letrozole is relatively new and it may may take some time before it is routinely used as the fertility world is so familiar with clomifene.

metformin

The theory behind the use of metformin for fertility follows the notion that it is testosterone within the ovary that applies the brakes to the maturing follicle so that ovulation is delayed. Metformin, by reducing the amount of insulin in the circulation, in turn reduces the amount of testosterone made within the ovary and therefore should allow eggs to be released in a more timely fashion. Certainly, some women who take metformin notice that periods are more regular. Just after the introduction of metformin in the 1990s it was thought that this treatment would be a breakthrough answer for many women who failed to ovulate with PCOS. It was not until about 2004 that well-constructed scientific research using the gold standard *randomised controlled trials* finally showed that metformin had no significant effect on improving fertility rates.

This is a curious turn of events – if periods are more regular then why is fertility not improved with Metformin? The explanation for this discrepancy between clinical experience and scientific research is that when metformin is used, it is usually combined with lifestyle measures such as a careful diet and increased exercise. In fact, it appears that it is the lifestyle change that brings about the improved fertility and not metformin itself (and here is a lesson that it is our own efforts to improve health that are most important, and there is no simple drug prescription that bypasses this discipline).

Despite the scientific research, there are some situations where metformin may still be used in a fertility setting. First, there are those women with oligomenorrhoea who may be a year or two away from the time when they plan to start a family. Metformin might give the edge to a lifestyle programme to allow a regular menstrual cycle to kick in a little earlier than might be expected with lifestyle measures alone. Second, in IVF treatment there is clear scientific evidence showing that adding metformin to a treatment programme reduces the chance of the side effect of ovarian hyperstimulation syndrome.

The main point to remember about metformin is that it is not a first-line treatment for fertility – for ovulation induction clomifene wins every time.

LH and FSH – the gonadotrophins

If ovulation does not occur after clomifene then it is assumed that the ovaries are 'resistant' to this treatment. The next level of treatment is usually daily injections of gonadotrophins.

FSH is the main hormone that drives the maturing follicle and it can be given by daily injection. FSH for treatment is made in two ways. For many years the gonadotropins LH and FSH have been extracted in a very pure form from urine collected from women who had passed the menopause – hence the name – human menopausal gonadotrophin or hMG. After the menopause, levels of LH and FSH are running very high in the blood and a proportion appears in the urine. Although this sounds extraordinary, this is a very well established and perfectly safe treatment that has been tried and tested for over 50 years. More recently bacteria have been programmed in their genes to make this hormone – so called recombinant FSH or rFSH. For most practical purposes there is no difference between urinary extracted hMG and recombinant rFSH and the choice is made based on the experience of the clinic and price.

hMG is available in vials of dried hormone that are made up each day with liquid and then injected. rFSH is available in pen injector devices that have the benefit that fine dose adjustment can be made. The doses are defined in international units and the starting dose for each cycle is between 37.5 and 75 iu.

Treatment starts soon after the beginning of a period and progress is monitored by using a series of ultrasound scans starting on about day seven after the first injection and then again at intervals every few days. At each scan appointment the number of follicles is carefully counted and the size of the largest one is compared to the previous scan so that the rate of growth can be plotted. The size of follicles at the start of treatment is about 5 mm and these grow to over 20 mm at the time of ovulation. Monitoring of injection treatment is a little more intensive compared to clomifene because the entire process is controlled by each dose adjustment on a day-by-day basis. For instance, a common treatment plan would be to start a cycle with 75 iu of hMG and increase to 100 iu after a week and then to 150 iu or even higher if the follicles are slow to grow.

When the lead or dominant follicle reaches about 20 mm an injection is given to release the egg. Human chorionic gonadotrophin or hCG is a hormone that works in the body like LH – the hormone that triggers ovulation. A single injection of hCG 5,000 to 10,000 units will release the egg. Intercourse, or intra-uterine insemination if it is being used, is best timed for about 36 hours after the hCG injection – the time it takes for the egg to travel down the fallopian tube.

The success of ovulation can be determined by a measurement of blood levels of progesterone and an ultrasound scan one week after ovulation. About two thirds of women who do not respond to clomifene will conceive with hMG. If ovulation does not happen then the treatment cycle is reviewed to see if there is any way to make the regimen more effective. If it is felt that hMG treatment is not going to work then the next level of treatment is planned.

ovarian diathermy or drilling

Ovarian diathermy or drilling is a type of fertility treatment that is popular in some clinics but many others may skip this step. This treatment requires a general anaesthetic for a laparoscope to be passed through the tummy button so that each ovary can be approached in turn. With a heating device called a diathermy probe, small burns are made on the surface of each ovary. For reasons that are poorly understood, this small amount of irritation to the ovary is sufficient to encourage regular ovulation for many months to follow.

Ovarian diathermy was a natural progression from an old operation that was performed in the 1950s. Because polycystic ovaries were slightly enlarged, it occurred to surgeons that removing a wedge from the ovary would correct the defect. For many years the operation called *wedge resection* was undertaken with moderate success. The damage caused to the ovary seems to bring about a regular cycle and some women became pregnant after this procedure. However, it was very difficult to fine-tune the amount of damage inflicted, so on some occasions the ovaries were damaged resulting in ovarian failure or early menopause. In addition, inflammation at the site of the cut on the surface of the ovary could cause the ovary to stick in an unfavourable position within the pelvis. Such pelvic adhesions might prevent the egg from jumping the distance between the ovary and the end of the fallopian tube.

Over the years the procedure was refined. It was found that simply four small burns would do the trick. The procedure has been extensively studied and there is very little risk of significant damage to the ovary or of adhesions that might affect fertility. The reason why ovarian diathermy is not used in some clinics is that it requires a general anaesthetic and a minor laparoscopic procedure. On the other hand, if laparoscopy is required for another reason for a woman with PCOS, such as to inspect the extent of endometriosis, then ovarian diathermy could be performed at the same time with no additional risk.

After ovarian diathermy approximately three quarters of women will change from having very irregular periods to having a predictable monthly cycle and they will be able to conceive without any further assistance. If regular periods do not return within three to four months then ovulation induction could be tried again starting with clomifene. That is, if somebody was previously clomifene-resistant before diathermy then it would be worth returning to clomifene again as it may begin to work after this procedure.

in vitro fertilisation – IVF

IVF is the most intensive treatment of all. It is the option if all attempts at ovulation induction have been unsuccessful. IVF is used for many causes of infertility such as blocked fallopian tubes or very low sperm count.

One part of the fertility process that can only be tested using IVF is the ability of the sperm to fertilise the egg. Instead of fertilisation taking place within the womb, the egg and sperm are combined in a test-tube so that fertilisation can be observed under a microscope – hence the old-fashioned term of a *test-tube baby*. IVF also has the benefit of selecting the best embryo from a batch of eggs instead of taking a chance with one egg each month using ovulation induction. Clinics will quote success rates for the chances of pregnancy ranging from 30% to 60% per cycle depending on the skill of the laboratory and, of course, the age of the mother.

The whole process of IVF is completely different from ovulation induction. With IVF, the ovary is first switched off by suppressing LH and FSH with a procedure called *down-regulation*. Down-regulation is achieved with highly potent versions of a small hormone called gonadotrophin-releasing hormone or GnRH analogues. GnRH analogues switch off the pituitary so that the ovary goes completely to sleep with no stimulation from LH and FSH. Injections of hMG are then started in a similar fashion to that described in ovulation induction except at higher doses because the overall object is to promote many eggs all at once. When the eggs are ripe, that is over 20 mm in size, they are removed from the ovary via a small needle placed through the side wall of the vagina. This procedure takes place either under anaesthetic or under sedation. As many as 20 or 30 eggs may be harvested in this way. In women with low ovarian reserve however, only a few eggs may be retrieved.

Once the eggs are available they are each placed in a different dish and are combined with a sample of sperm to allow fertilisation. The egg and sperm are kept in an incubator for several days while they begin to grow and subsequently can be seen to divide. The healthiest amongst the embryos are then transferred into the uterus in the hope that they will implant. In the early days of IVF several embryos were put back but this meant there was a risk of having twins or triplets. Nowadays, it is advised that only one embryo or at most two embryos are put back in order to reduce the risk of multiple pregnancy.

The exact treatment programme for IVF will vary from clinic to clinic and it is beyond the scope of this book to present more than an overview of the whole procedure.

One of the most important risks involved in IVF treatment is that of driving the ovaries too hard so that they are stimulated to enlarge to the point where they cause discomfort – perhaps measuring 10 cm instead of 3 cm. This is a condition called *ovarian hyperstimulation syndrome* or OHSS. As clinics have become more and more skilled at controlling this hormone treatment, so the number of women experiencing OHSS has declined over the years. Nevertheless, women with PCOS are very sensitive to this hormone treatment. In PCOS, the line between producing sufficient eggs for success yet holding back to stop OHSS is very thin. In the most severe cases of OHSS, admission into hospital is required for close observation and treatment.

summary of fertility and PCOS

Overall, taking all of the treatment options into account, the chances of having children for women with PCOS is normal.

Simple tablet treatment with clomifene will usually be the answer if periods are infrequent and IVF is rarely required.

Women with PCOS do not necessarily have to start a family any earlier than average. However, for all women fertility success declines after the age of 38 and in the UK no fertility treatment is offered in the NHS over the age of 40. For women who are overweight early pre-pregnancy planning is important not only to make getting pregnant easier, but also to ensure a healthy pregnancy free of complication – especially diabetes.

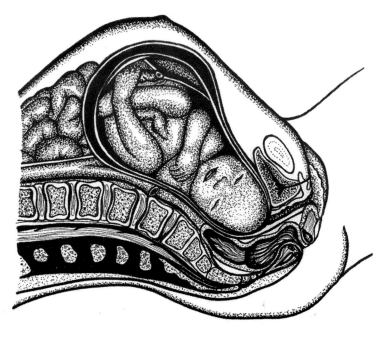

a baby in utero

In this picture, the baby is within the uterus with the placenta at the top of the picture. Below is the spinal cord of the mother. To the left are the intestines, to the right is the vagina with the bladder above, and above that the pelvis bone.

chapter 7
preparing for pregnancy

The first three months of pregnancy can often be the most worrying time because of the risk of miscarriage.

Whether pregnancy was achieved easily without medical assistance or fertility treatment was required, the mind turns to problems that might arise as pregnancy proceeds. Quite a lot has been written about how women with PCOS might have more problems in pregnancy. Some of the contributors have tended to exaggerate some of the risks. The reason for this is that many studies have looked only at women who are receiving fertility treatment. This group of women is known to have higher risks in pregnancy compared to women who fall pregnant spontaneously. Also, women who go through fertility treatment tend to be older than average which can account for some of the higher risks of pregnancy.

For those women who have received fertility treatment, a pregnancy is particularly precious. It is certainly worth looking at all of the areas that might improve health in pregnancy when preparing to start a family.

is the risk of miscarriage higher in PCOS?

There is quite a lot of information on the Internet suggesting that women with PCOS have a higher risk of miscarriage than average. In fact the scientific evidence to support this is very weak. That is to say, it is unlikely that PCOS alone carries any extra risk of miscarriage.

It is well known that older women and those who are overweight have a higher risk of miscarriage than average. When you look at all of the papers describing a higher risk of miscarriage in PCOS, differences disappear when the effect of excess weight is taken into account. Similarly, if you come across papers describing a high risk of miscarriage in PCOS, you need to look very carefully at whether comparison groups are of similar age.

In conclusion, PCOS probably has no extra risk of miscarriage attached to it but the issue regarding overweight is important. Weight loss is one of the only factors related to miscarriage that you can alter before getting pregnant. Therefore, if time allows, a weight-loss programme for six months leading up to pregnancy would be sensible as outlined below.

Other misleading information on the Internet suggests that metformin might lower the risk of miscarriage. These reports started to appear in the 1990s as soon as metformin began to be used in PCOS. A clinic might report that before it started using metformin, 20 per cent of pregnancies resulted in miscarriage whereas after that the figure was only 10 percent. The scientific error committed by these papers was failing to report that other things had happened at the same time as introducing metformin. Most importantly, women taking metformin were likely to have taken on a change in diet and an increase in exercise. These lifestyle changes probably account for the reduced miscarriage rate. Later studies, which use the more rigorous design of a *randomised controlled trial*, showed no effect of metformin on the risk of miscarriage. For this reason, it is advised that women should stop taking metformin as soon as they find they are pregnant. It simply has no benefit in early pregnancy unless diabetes is the issue.

am I likely to get diabetes in pregnancy?

As women with PCOS are more likely to be overweight with insulin resistance in the family, the risk of diabetes in pregnancy may be increased. Diabetes in pregnancy is an important problem because if the mother runs a high blood sugar then the fetus can grow too big. This can cause complications in childbirth and might even cause a higher risk of diabetes for the baby later in life.

Diabetes in pregnancy is called *gestational diabetes mellitus* (GDM). It is checked for routinely in the antenatal clinic. Every woman, whether they have PCOS or not, will be checked in pregnancy with a blood glucose test. If the blood sugar level is higher than average then the antenatal doctors may request an oral glucose tolerance test to see how the body handles a sugar drink with blood glucose tested two hours later (see chapter 2).

Most of the papers recording a higher risk of gestational diabetes in PCOS share the problems to those reporting miscarriage. Those that were very carefully matched for weight sometimes found that there was no excess risk of diabetes in pregnancy for women with PCOS. Therefore, reports that the rate of gestational diabetes in pregnancy may be 10 times greater in women with PCOS overestimate the problem. The only paper that can be considered accurate on this subject states the risk of GDM as 2.3 times greater for women with PCOS compared to controls. This came from a study of over 3700 women with PCOS in Sweden. GMD is estimated to affect 10% of pregnancies in the UK, so for women with PCOS this figure might go up to 23% – nearly a quarter of all women. This reference can be found in chapter 11.

Another type of study that has been undertaken is checking for whether women who have gestational diabetes are more likely than average to have polycystic ovaries on ultrasound. These studies are all in general agreement that there is an overlap between gestational diabetes and polycystic ovaries.

Diabetes in pregnancy can be an early warning of the risk of acquiring type 2 diabetes later in life. The big risk of becoming diabetic is if you have a parent with diabetes. Linking these two points for women with PCOS; if you have a parent with diabetes then you should consider yourself to be at risk of gestational diabetes. It would be advisable to be extra careful with your diet from the outset of pregnancy or even before. A family history of diabetes is probably a more important point that any amount of testing for blood sugar.

In conclusion, women with PCOS, particularly those who have received fertility treatment, have a slightly higher rate of diabetes in pregnancy that is mainly related to being overweight. The risk of gestational diabetes can be reduced in two ways; trying to achieve an average body weight before conceiving and by keeping to a careful healthy low-carbohydrate diet with no refined sugar during pregnancy.

what about high blood pressure in pregnancy?

As well as measuring blood sugar and the size of the baby, the other potential problem checked for in antenatal clinics is blood pressure. Blood pressure tends to go up in the last three months of pregnancy. There is a risk that this can turn into a serious medical problem called *pre-eclampsia*.

Until recently the scientific papers were not clear on whether pre-eclampsia was more common in PCOS than average. The situation has been clarified recently with the same paper from Sweden that clarified the diabetes risk. This paper reported that the risk of pre-eclampsia is increased by about 50 percent in women with PCOS.

Why blood pressure and pre-eclampsia are more common in PCOS is unknown. One possibility is that some of the substances made by the ovary might affect blood pressure. For instance, polycystic ovaries make more than the average amount of a substance called *vascular endothelial growth factor* or VEGF that might constrict the blood vessels in a way that puts up the blood pressure. At the time of writing, all of this is conjecture that needs to be explored.

I may want to get pregnant in a year's time – what should I be doing now?

There are entire books on the subject of getting healthy before pregnancy. Any number of multivitamin preparations are sold for this indication. It is always worthwhile taking stock of all health issues by seeing your GP for a pre-conception talk. Some advice such as taking folic acid is now becoming routine. Other pieces of advice are not so well tested and might follow a fashion rather than science. Your GP will also go through any drugs that you are taking to see if they are OK in pregnancy. With some drugs we have quite a lot of information on their safety in pregnancy but with others, especially the new ones, there can be no safety data. If in doubt, aim to be as drug-free as possible for the weeks leading up to pregnancy.

There are some important topics to cover that relate specifically to women with PCOS, taking into account the risks of pregnancy that are outlined above.

if I stop my treatment to get pregnant will all of my problems come back?

Obviously, you will have to come off the pill before getting pregnant! Before doing so however, there should be a plan about anti-androgen treatment. For women who know that their acne or hirsutism can return very quickly if they stop treatment, there can be anxiety about how they will fare in the window between having to stop treatment and conceiving. Rather than stop the pill and spironolactone together, they can be phased out making the treatment-free time as short as possible. Usually the anti-androgen is stopped first and then the pill is stopped three months later.

Any treatment that interferes with the action of testosterone such as cyproterone acetate or spironolactone, could have a bad effect on the early development of a boy. Testosterone made by the male fetus will control how the penis develops. This is not an area where you would want to take any chances! It is generally advised that you stop anti-androgens for three months before conceiving. During these three months you may want to continue with the pill so that you do not have a chance of getting pregnant too quickly while these drugs wear out of the system. In addition, the pill will help to keep any symptoms such as acne or hirsutism at bay. In the anti-androgen family of drugs it is finasteride that is thought to be the most serious for affecting a baby so this one in particular has to be stopped well ahead of time.

It is helpful to know what to expect for a period pattern. Some women who have been on the pill for many years will not be able to predict this with any certainty. The point here is that if oligomenorrhoea is likely to return then it may not be sensible to wait a whole year before seeking fertility advice. You could start tests to see if you ovulate after three months have passed which is the minimum time allowed for periods to settle after using the pill. In this way it might be possible to shorten the time when acne may return. Once pregnant, the ovaries go to sleep so acne and hirsutism are rarely a problem until the end of breastfeeding.

There are some drugs relating to PCOS that have been used routinely as fertility treatments. These are considered safe to take even if you get pregnant while taking them. This list includes metformin, clomifene, gonadotrophins, thyroxine, progesterone and drugs that lower prolactin. With regard to the progesterone family, it is thought that the stronger synthetic types such as norethisterone and medroxyprogesterone might increase the risk of an ectopic pregnancy whereas natural progesterone that is used in IVF fertility treatments is OK.

with my PCOS, do I need a blood test before trying to get pregnant?

There are some routine tests worth having prior to pregnancy even though they are not closely related to PCOS and are not always performed in routine practice.

Blood sugar – Most women with PCOS get pregnant without having any special blood test before. However, because of the risk of diabetes in pregnancy it might be advisable for some women with PCOS to run some tests. For instance, if you have a family history of type 2 diabetes, if you know that your mother had diabetes in pregnancy or if you are overweight, then it would be worth considering an oral glucose tolerance test. An OGTT will establish the risk of getting diabetes. The result will also alert you as to how far you might have to go with diet and exercise to reduce this risk.

Thyroid – An underactive thyroid gland is quite common, affecting up to three percent of women. Hypothyroidism is associated with a higher than average risk of miscarriage. Thyroid deficiency is also thought to be more common in PCOS. Together, these two observations make a thyroid function test worthwhile. Recent research shows that the level of thyroid function should be adjusted precisely in early pregnancy to reduce the associated miscarriage risk. The level of thyroid function is best measured by a test for *thyroid stimulating hormone* or TSH. The reference range for TSH is usually something like 0.3 to 5.0 iu/L with levels above this indicating an underactive thyroid gland. Some authorities recommend moving the goal posts for women who want to conceive to make a reference range of 0.3 to 2.5 iu/L. The lower value at the top of the reference range means that some women will need to take a supplement of thyroid hormone to achieve this. This area is relatively new so we only have preliminary trials to go by. As we learn more this advice may change over coming years. Also, you may find that doctors disagree on whether it is a good idea to take thyroxine if it is not strictly necessary.

Vitamins and Minerals – If you have been prone to very heavy periods then a very mild level of iron deficiency might be present. For iron status the best screening test is *serum ferritin*. You should aim to get your level into the upper half of the normal range as insurance against anaemia in pregnancy. Your baby will be taking some of your iron when it starts making its own blood cells. By the same token, mild vitamin D deficiency is common in the UK because of relatively low light exposure the further north you get. There is a fashion for taking vitamin D supplements. While we do not have any scientific proof that this is a benefit in pregnancy, it is a simple natural substance that might assist you in absorbing calcium that will eventually make its way to your baby. Vitamin D can be simply measured on a blood test but just taking a low dose supplement such as vitamin D 25 mcg (the same as 1000 units) should do the job. While multivitamins may contain both iron and vitamin D, they often contain too little to really increase the levels in the blood stream if your starting point is low. It might be worthwhile taking these two supplements separately. Vitamin B_{12} is reported to run low in women who have taken metformin for many months. Most pregnancy multivitamins provide sufficient support for vitamin B_{12} but if in doubt, a blood test is available.

what can I do to lower the risk of complications in pregnancy?

Before trying to get pregnant it is worthwhile thinking about how to reduce the risks of complications in pregnancy with a particular focus on diabetes and blood pressure. If you are overweight, losing weight can reduce the risk of diabetes. If you are of normal weight however, trying to drive yourself down to the lower range of BMI probably has no benefit. Indeed, low body weight may make it more difficult to get pregnant. It is possible to stop ovulating simply by having a very calorie-restricted diet or by losing weight if you are already at the lower end of the normal range.

All of the issues relating to a healthy diet become more important before and during pregnancy. This is a time to be particularly strict about eliminating all sugars in the diet, eating natural foods and reducing the portions of refined carbohydrate.

With regard to blood pressure, the main component in the diet that will affect this is salt. Like sugar, salt is found in many commercially produced foods. Salt is an unnecessary part of the diet. By making you retain more fluid in the circulation, excess salt can raise blood pressure. It is estimated that you can reduce the blood pressure by five points (mmHg) by introducing a low-salt diet. While it may be that only one in 20 women with PCOS run into trouble with high blood pressure in pregnancy, it seems sensible to try to prevent becoming one of these five percent. As in all things, prevention is better than cure.

further reading

There is only one really good scientific paper that looks at complications in pregnancy for women with PCOS:

Risk of adverse pregnancy outcomes in women with polycystic ovary syndrome: population based cohort study. Nathalie Roos et al British Medical Journal 2011 – see chapter 11.

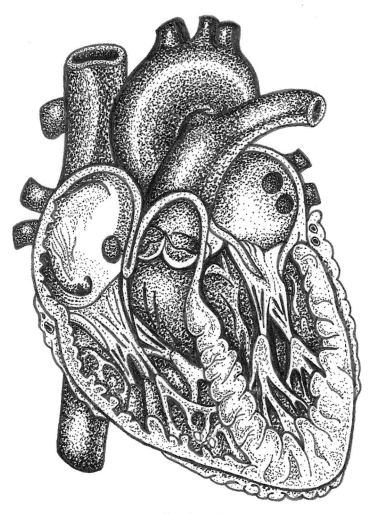

the heart

This picture shows the two ventricles of the heart – right and left – opened up so that the muscles that control the heart valves can be seen. At the top of the picture is the aortic arch that will deliver blood around the body. The vessel running above and below on the left is the vena cava which is bringing blood in to the heart after it has circulated around the body.

chapter 8
long-term health issues

It can be alarming to be labeled with a new diagnosis for the first time. Not only do you have to think about the immediate effects of a condition but you also have to take on board possible implications for long-term health. Most healthy young people never question their mortality but as soon as a diagnosis is made, inevitably the mind turns to future well-being. Happily, extensive research has shown that there are few surprises in store for someone with PCOS as they grow older.

Briefly, there is an increased tendency to develop type 2 diabetes. There has been some debate about whether there is an increased risk of heart disease but research so far indicates that this is not the case. These aspects will be covered in more detail later in the chapter.

what happens to polycystic ovaries after the menopause?

The average age of the menopause, which is between 50 and 51 years of age, is no different for women with PCOS than in the general population. In the years leading up to the menopause you would expect that many of the symptoms would improve as the level of testosterone in all women (and in men too!) gradually declines with age. As the number of follicles in the ovary declines with age, so the amount of testosterone made also come down. Having said this, there are very few research studies that have followed the natural history of PCOS for more than a few years. It is not clear how the ultrasound picture of polycystic ovaries changes over time. It may be that the polycystic ovary change never completely disappears until the time of the menopause. There have been attempts to describe how polycystic ovaries appear on ultrasound in women after the menopause but the outcome of these studies have not provided a clear conclusion of whether the ovaries continue to look different from women who never had PCOS.

We have some knowledge of what happens to the symptoms of PCOS over years. The interval between periods tends to get shorter as the menopause approaches. Many women with PCOS who have very infrequent periods in their 20s, turn out to have a regular menstrual cycle in their 40s. On the other hand, symptoms such as hirsutism and acne do not seem to improve greatly over time.

The balance of testosterone and oestrogen in the body takes an interesting course in the menopause. The most dramatic hormone change that occurs at the menopause is the lower oestrogen levels that give rise to the classical symptoms. The fall in testosterone that should occur in parallel with oestrogen is relatively less. In this way, the balance of testosterone and oestrogen at the time of the menopause slightly favours an excess of testosterone. This testosterone effect at the menopause is the reason why many women experience unwanted hair growth after the menopause, whether you have PCOS or not. It is likely that if hair follicles have been driven by high testosterone throughout life then the effect of testosterone at the menopause will be more pronounced. In other words, women with PCOS may experience more unwanted hair growth at menopause than average.

Treatments of unwanted hair growth at the menopause differ from those used in young life. For instance, it is not recommended to use the combined oral contraceptive pill in your 40s and 50s. Instead, treatment will be based on anti-androgens such as spironolactone and topical treatments such as Vaniqa.

should I use HRT after the menopause?

The need for *hormone replacement therapy* (HRT) at the menopause is the same for women with PCOS as for those without. HRT is mainly needed for those women who have prominent symptoms of the lack of oestrogen such as hot flushes, disturbed sleep, panic attacks and brain fog. The symptoms usually last for a few years while the body adjusts to lower oestrogen levels.

There is a spectrum of experience of symptoms related to the menopause. Some women barely detect the change in hormone levels. They would never need to think about taking HRT. At the other end of the spectrum are those who have such severe symptoms that they would never consider coming off HRT. If HRT is used for over five years, there is a slightly increased risk of breast cancer. It is a personal choice whether this increased cancer risk is acceptable when balanced against improved quality of life in the short-term. At a practical level, routine breast examination and mammograms should be sufficient precaution to allow continued use of HRT.

With regard to women with PCOS, oestrogen contained within most HRT formulations may have an added benefit by helping to suppress unwanted hair growth. This factor has to be taken into account when weighing up the pros and cons of HRT for each individual.

will my weight finally behave itself after the menopause?

If it was that the ovaries were the driving force to weight gain then you would expect that after the menopause difficulty with weight control would no longer be a problem. Unfortunately, things are never that simple – especially when weight loss is concerned. Polycystic ovaries are not the cause for overweight so this fervent hope will not come true. Overweight and polycystic ovaries are inherited separately. It is the experience of many women that the metabolism does not change much at the time of the menopause. In fact, women tend to gain weight around the waist as a result of oestrogen deficiency. There is no increase in the metabolic rate at this time. Also, the basal metabolic rate falls with age, which adds to the tendency for women to gain weight in their 50s.

is my risk of cancer higher because I have PCOS?

The important cancer risk that was first discussed in chapter 4, is cancer of the lining of the womb – endometrial cancer. Women who are overweight and who have had infrequent periods may develop an excessive thickening of the lining of the womb called *endometrial hyperplasia*. This develops because the lining is never shed completely. As periods are far apart, the endometrium grows thicker and thicker with the risk of becoming organised as a group of cells that are at risk of cancer.

Endometrial hyperplasia is easily detected on an ultrasound where a thickness of between 12 and 25 mm may be seen instead of the usual measurement of less than 10 mm. The general guideline is that endometrial hyperplasia should not be a problem as long as you have at least four periods per year. Some specialists however, prefer to play on the safe side and recommend <u>monthly</u> periods. For women with very infrequent periods, withdrawal bleeds have to be induced using either an oral contraceptive pill or cyclical progesterone (see chapter 4).

There are no other cancers that are more common for women with PCOS. Some researchers have questioned whether breast cancer might be more common but in fact there is no good evidence that this is so. Similarly there is no increased risk of cancer of the ovary for women with PCOS.

what is my risk of getting diabetes later in life?

Because of the discussion about insulin resistance in PCOS there has been some concern about the risk of developing type 2 diabetes. Some people have considered PCOS to be a forerunner of diabetes or a *pre-diabetic* state. Put in the terms of a lifetime, some women who present with PCOS in their 20s or 30s may then go on to develop type 2 diabetes. If we could predict who might follow this route then we could work hard at an early stage to prevent diabetes with lifestyle changes. In fact, having PCOS is not as important a risk factor for diabetes compared to the two front-runners: family history and bodyweight.

Type 2 diabetes is strongly inherited – much more so than the younger group who require insulin injections with type I diabetes. Type I diabetes is a completely different process that is not related to PCOS. If you have one parent with type 2 diabetes it is estimated that you have a 50% risk of also acquiring it. If you have two parents with type 2 diabetes then your risk of also getting it may be as high as 80%. Although some genes have been identified that can predict this risk, genetic testing is not available routinely as the genes described so far only account for a small proportion of the risk.

Type 2 diabetes is caused primarily by the body being unable to keep up an adequate insulin supply to overcome insulin resistance. Insulin resistance in turn, is brought about mainly by overweight. The tendency to develop diabetes as a result of weight gain is the main reason why obesity is a health risk. In other words, it is mainly because of diabetes that life expectancy is reduced in someone who is overweight. By losing weight, the action of insulin in the body improves. In fact, mild diabetes can be completely reversed with diet and exercise.

Interestingly, a diabetes prevention study performed in Finland compared using diet and exercise to long-term treatment with metformin as a method of preventing diabetes in high-risk people. Diet and exercise turned out to be twice as effective as metformin. This study acts as a reminder that we cannot rely on a simple tablet to replace hard work and willpower for improved metabolism.

If you have a parent with type 2 diabetes and you are overweight then you have the two major risk factors for getting diabetes yourself. It is important to seek early medical advice. If you have a first-degree relative with diabetes, are overweight and you have PCOS then you have a full house of risk factors even though the PCOS is the lesser of the three. The most extensive long-term health study for women with PCOS showed that after 31 years the extra risk of diabetes was accounted for by overweight.

The capacity of the body to make insulin declines with age, so getting older is another risk factor for type 2 diabetes. Having said that, there is now great concern that type 2 diabetes, which always used to be a condition of older people, is now appearing in teenagers because of the epidemic of obesity.

with PCOS, will my risk of heart disease go up?

Heart disease is the most common cause of death for all women but no more so in women with PCOS than average. This fact is based mainly on a follow-up of women with PCOS over 30 years. There are many papers that report that the risk of heart disease should be higher in women with PCOS because of risk factors such as a bad cholesterol profile. This turns out not to be the case in long-term studies. How can we resolve this discrepancy?

The three main risk factors for heart disease that are commonly found in women with PCOS are excess weight, diabetes and an adverse cholesterol profile. Women with diabetes lose the protection of being female as they have the same risk of heart disease as men – that is quite a big risk difference. Overall, overweight is such a strong influence on heart disease risk that it is hard to separate out an independent risk related to PCOS itself.

While this research can reassure us, we must remember that the information was collected in the past so conclusions on heart disease risk may not apply to the future. For instance, the most influential study focused on women who had PCOS in the 1950s and 1960s which was a time when our lifestyles were better than they are now. In those days, everyone took more exercise and had a healthier diet. We have yet to see how the epidemic of obesity will impact on future health. It may be that women with PCOS will only show the extra heart disease risk when they have been overweight for a substantial time in their lives. Unfortunately we are always working thirty years behind in our assessment of mortality risk.

There is another challenging theory as to why women with PCOS can have a higher risk of diabetes but not heart disease. It may be that polycystic ovaries actually <u>protects</u> from heart disease to some degree. It may be only the women without PCOS who develop type 2 diabetes that have the higher incidence of heart disease. It is conceivable that some factor made by the ovary improves blood flow to the heart without affecting the action of insulin. Here we enter the realm of conjecture!

what about high blood pressure?

High blood pressure is important because it leads to life-threatening heart attacks and stroke. Inside the heart, a heart attack occurs when the blood flow to a segment of muscle is blocked. This muscle subsequently dies. As a result, the heart is weaker. It can be that a heart attack is so overwhelming that there is simply not enough muscle to continue the pump action. This is why a heart attack is a common cause of sudden death. The lead up to a heart attack, or in medical terms a *myocardial infarction*, is a combination of two processes. First, the arteries of the heart begin to get clogged up with patches of cholesterol that become inflamed – hardening of the arteries. Second, a blood clot forms over the inflamed inner lining of the artery blocking the flow of blood – everything downstream of the blockage dies.

High blood pressure or *hypertension* is a related condition as it can lead to a heart attack or heart failure. The risk of high blood pressure is increased in obesity because high pressures are required in order to pump blood around a bigger body. High blood pressure is related to PCOS but the relationship is mainly accounted for by excess weight. High blood pressure in pregnancy is related to PCOS so it may well be that there is a background tendency to high blood pressure that we need to look out for as a woman with PCOS grows older.

A blood pressure check is a routine part of any medical check-up and after the age of fifty it should be checked. Blood pressure treatments are now so effective with so few side-effects that it is always better to start treatment early in a preventative way rather than to hold off taking tablets for as long as possible.

High blood pressure is a side-effect of taking a combined oral contraceptive which is commonly used in young women with PCOS. Everyone taking the pill should have a blood pressure check taken every six months – usually with each new prescription. If blood pressure becomes a problem then the pill has to be stopped. It is usually possible to find alternatives to the pill if necessary.

is the thyroid gland related to PCOS?

An underactive thyroid gland – *hypothyroidism* – is a common condition that affects about 3% of women. It would not be unusual therefore, for hypothyroidism and PCOS to occur at the same time. A blood test for thyroid hormones is often included on a routine screen as part of a work-up for PCOS. There are several reports that an underactive thyroid gland is more common in PCOS than in the general population. It is not certain why this should be. Women who have an underactive thyroid gland tend to gain weight. This might be the link to why this problem is commonly found in women with PCOS.

The treatment for an overactive thyroid gland is very simple. Thyroxine is available by routine prescription. It is used in the same way for women with PCOS as for all other women with hypothyroidism.

osteoporosis runs in my family, will PCOS make it worse?

There is no link between PCOS and osteoporosis. There is often some confusion about a possible link between these two conditions. This confusion comes about because there is a connection between other causes of a lack of periods (amenorrhoea) and osteoporosis. In all other causes of amenorrhoea, oestrogen levels are low. This is a cause of bone loss. PCOS is the one of the few causes of amenorrhoea where oestrogen levels are normal so there should be no excess risk of osteoporosis.

Everyone reaches their peak bone mass between the ages of 25 and 35. This is when the bones are at their strongest. Thereafter, everybody loses 1% to 2% of bone every year. The most important hormone in the body that contributes to bone strength is oestrogen. Oestrogen helps strengthen the protein matrix upon which calcium is laid down in bone. Women who are lacking oestrogen early in their lives have a high risk of osteoporosis later in life.

There has been some concern that treatments that block testosterone could have a bad effect on bone. Testosterone has some bone-building action, but this is less important compared to the effect of oestrogen. Theoretically, therefore, an anti-testosterone treatment such as cyproterone acetate or spironolactone could be a risk for osteoporosis. Spironolactone however has both anti-testosterone and oestrogen-like properties that probably cancel each other out so this treatment has no effect on bone. Cyproterone acetate on the other hand tends to lower oestrogen levels in the body. Also, it has a slight steroid-like effect which could be a risk for osteoporosis. This risk probably only applies to women taking reasonably high-dose treatment such as 25 mg per day or above for many years.

summary

In conclusion, although this chapter lists a number of conditions that have come up for discussion as women with PCOS enter middle age, it is only diabetes and high blood pressure that show up consistently. It is well worth being aware of the family history for both of these conditions. Think about getting checked at an early stage if either run through the family.

It is a curious thing that the risk factors for heart disease do not seem to materialise as actual heart attacks in women with PCOS. This is an area where we need more research to understand the links better.

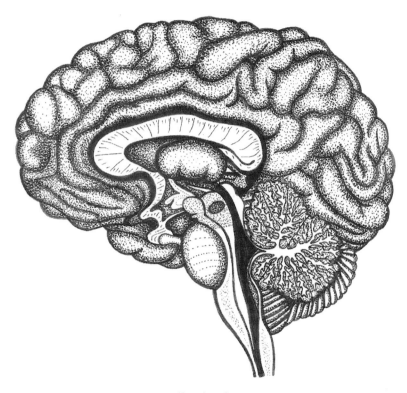

the brain

The main part of the brain is the cortex that looks like a bag of sausages around the top surface. Below this is the corpus callosum that joins the two sides of the brain together. The cabbage-like structure on the right-hand side is the cerebellum – the center for coordination in the brain. Extending downwards is the spinal cord.

chapter 9

lifestyle, alternative therapies and diet

So far, the content of this book has come from experience in hospital-based clinics using a conventional medical management. This approach was adopted in response to comments from patients that such information is difficult to access. It is obvious however, that conventional medicine offers no 'cure' for women with PCOS. In many ways, the standard treatments are limited in that they fail to completely resolve the symptoms. Other types of therapy have an important place for women with PCOS. Often, the key to moving forward is to abandon the notion of there being a perfect fix. Instead, well-being comes from taking control of the problem.

Feeling empowered to take ownership of PCOS is often a difficult first step. Many of the topics covered in this chapter have the aim of improving self-confidence in the hope that this will enable women to conquer the difficulties related to PCOS – particularly with weight control. *Patient empowerment* is a buzzword in health care but how to achieve it is another matter. The idea is to move from external pressure ('my doctor says I should lose weight') to the more positive internal motivation ('losing weight is really important for me').

It is very hard to know which therapy would be best for you. There are many books on alternative therapies but little guidance on how to compare one with another. It is impossible to properly compare alternative treatments because they are not standardised and many of the outcomes are subjective. Each woman has to feel her way with different options. The choice of therapy may be based on those that one has the greatest natural faith in, a therapy that comes recommended or because of a particularly good personal approach by the therapist. It may be a case of trial and error in the first instance. A good therapist in almost any field may help build a positive way forward.

Browsing the Internet is a difficult way to judge the effectiveness of a therapy as self-promotion makes any service seem great. No one advertises failures! Support groups and forums, where real-life experiences can be shared, are a good bet.

This chapter will touch upon topics that have come up in discussion either in clinic or at support group meetings. It must be emphasised however, that this is not a definitive list nor does any one form of therapy come with a personal recommendation.

exercise

The general advice on exercise for everyone (PCOS or not!) is to achieve a 20–30 minute session three times per week. Of course, if you do more, then you get extra benefit. The best type of exercise is the one that makes you happy – so that you are likely to keep up with it! It is not necessary to become too academic about the relative merits of different systems – choose something that you like. Cardiovascular exercise has benefits of burning calories. Isometric or weight-based exercise gives additional improvement in insulin sensitivity. Start small, and then build up so that the exercise becomes sustainable.

For cardiovascular exercise the key is to push the pace so that the pulse rate goes up over 120 beats per minute. Some advisors favour longer sessions of modest intensity over short bursts of intense exercise. The idea with this is that the body burns mainly stored *glycogen* for the first 20 minutes of exercise. After that it begins to burn fat tissue. It is the burning of fat tissue that seems to improve metabolic rate. Studies have shown that the metabolic rate is increased for some hours after such exercise although the scientific evidence for this shows the effect to be quite small unless you push for intensive prolonged exercise.

While membership to a gym is popular with some, it is certainly not essential or even the best option for others. There are additional benefits from being outside in the sun. Outdoor exercise may be better for both mood and the ability to stick to exercise. Long walks at the weekend, particularly with a walking group, are a popular option. For animal lovers, think about getting a dog to take on regular walks. Another sociable option is dancing – Zumba your way to regular periods!

A common recommendation is to try to achieve 10,000 steps per day. Simply by wearing a pedometer you can begin to see how sedentary your life is. Using a pedometer can be an encouragement to building a walk into everyday life. For instance, try walking to the shops at every opportunity instead of driving or choosing a more distant bus or underground station in your daily commute. A personal trainer may provide better discipline as an outside influence but at quite an expense.

iPCOS! – what's on the web?

In addition to support groups dedicated to PCOS, there are many web-based tools which *app*-enthusiasts might find useful. Some applications have the facility to bring together information from several users allowing an informal self-help group to work together.

There is a huge amount of information on the Internet regarding low glycaemic index diets or magical ways of removing abdominal fat! While most of this is a waste of time, some applications can be useful in learning about types of food. One example is 'myfitnesspal' that requires you to enter in your food intake so that you can see exactly what your calorie and sugar intake is. In addition, you can choose to set a low-carbohydrate content as a goal of your diet. The accumulated food data will remind you as you go through the day if you are in danger of exceeding this goal. Even if you are not sufficiently obsessive to keep this up on a daily basis, it can be very informative as a way of learning about your diet over a week or two. The idea is that such a system can help you change your food choices.

Activity monitors are becoming increasingly popular even though most are nothing more than a posh pedometer. If you are interested not only in counting how many calories go in but also in how many calories you burn, then you may find these helpful. The most popular are wristbands that usually synchronise with a web-based record of your daily activity. Some wristbands can also record your sleep pattern or connect to a heart rate monitor.

alternative therapies

cognitive behavioural therapy

CBT is not really an alternative therapy as it is widely used in mainstream medicine for conditions such as depression and fatigue. CBT is a type of talking therapy with sessions every week for at least six weeks – sometimes considerably longer. It also works well for weight loss. The effectiveness of this type of treatment is often better than most drug treatments. CBT practitioners may be found through primary care services.

In the younger age groups it is important to have someone outside of the family to contribute to goal setting rather than allow diet to become a point of conflict. When it comes to sticking to a lifestyle programme, positive reinforcement easily gives way to parents taking control in a negative way. It is really unfortunate that the symptoms of PCOS come on in adolescence at the same time as the common teenage issues relating to family dynamics and social relationships. Recognition of these interactions can be an essential part of success in overcoming the burden of PCOS for teenagers. This is where a counsellor, psychologist or behavioural therapist can be essential.

CBT is a considerable time commitment. It takes two or three sessions to design a personal programme. After that there are repeated one-hour sessions over six weeks to six months.

mindfullness

Mindfulness has its origin in Buddhist meditation focusing on the pattern of breathing. This practice has been adopted by psychologists who refined it into a form of cognitive therapy particularly for use in depression. Mindfulness is now popular in many clinical applications. It is also used in business to improve productivity.

Mindfulness meditation involves moment-by-moment awareness of thoughts, feelings and sensations. In this way, thought processes are focused on the senses and attention is drawn away from points of stress or sadness. By stopping the mind from dwelling on negative aspect of life, one can achieve an acceptance of the situation that hopefully leads to achieving positive goals in the future.

There are many courses for mindfulness on the market. While it has turned into something of a commercial business, it can be useful for the management of a life-long condition at a personal level.

nutritionist

A nutritionist can be a good lifestyle advisor as well as providing detailed meal planning. This approach can be good in the early phase of lifestyle changes when there might be a lot to take on in terms of changing diet. A nutritionist will also advise on vitamins and minerals but on the whole, with a healthy natural diet, additional vitamin supplements should not be required.

There is no specific length-of-time that nutritionist therapy should continue. It all depends on the type of role that the nutritionist takes on. Their input may be short-term education on food groups or it may be longer-term project management. The type of support will also depend on your starting point and how much dietary change you are planning to make. If you already have a healthy natural diet then a nutritionist may not have much to offer.

acupuncture

Acupuncture has many applications. From the scientific point of view, acupuncture is a logical approach as the signals from the pituitary to the ovary may well be changed by this method. It seems logical that acupuncture would work well for irregular periods that may in turn increase the reliability of ovulation.

Recently, scientific trials of using acupuncture for women with PCOS have reported a reduction in the blood concentration of androgens and an increase in the frequency of ovulation. These are promising initial results but whether every acupuncture therapist can achieve such a positive outcome is hard to say. In practice, acupuncture seems to be a useful 'add-on' treatment in conjunction with conventional therapy, perhaps as a way of improving the chance of a positive outcome to fertility treatment.

Speaking from first principles, acupuncture may not be so good for the long-term symptoms of unwanted hair growth or acne. New data on lower androgen concentrations with this treatment, however, makes this area of treatment a possibility to look out for in the future.

herbal medicine

There is a seemingly endless list of herbal supplements that might be beneficial for women with PCOS. None of the herbal remedies have good scientific evidence to support their use but several names come up on a regular basis. Rather than try supplements at random it might be worth seeking professional advice if a herbal approach is attractive to you. Mentioned here are a few that come up for discussion regularly.

Agnus Castus – some studies have shown that this treatment can lower prolactin leading indirectly to improved signalling from the pituitary to the ovary. This supplement has a reputation for reducing premenstrual symptoms, improving menstrual cycle control and fertility.

Black Cohosh – this supplement is thought to have some oestrogen-like activity. It may also act on serotonin receptors. Its reputation is for improving mood changes through the menstrual cycle.

Burdock root – the burdock plant or *Arctium* has thistle like flowers and its root can be used as a drink or applied to the skin for the treatment of acne.

Evening Primrose oil – this supplement contains a range of essential fatty acids including *gamma linolenic acid*. EPO has a reputation for improving premenstrual symptoms. Scientific trials are divided as to how successful this treatment is but anecdotally it has proved very popular.

Gingko biloba – this popular supplement has been used in a wide variety of conditions. It is thought to act through a variety of neuroendocrine receptors such as serotonin, dopamine and 5-HT. It may alter pituitary hormone signalling and therefore may be effective for premenstrual symptoms, period timing and ovulation.

Saw Palmetto – this herbal supplement it is of interest in lowering androgenic symptoms. Once again, scientific studies have failed to identify a real benefit. It is said to block the enzyme 5-alpha reductase which converts testosterone to dihydrotestosterone. Through this mechanism, one would expect this supplement to improve symptoms such as unwanted hair growth or acne.

Spearmint – tea made of Mentha spicata Labiatae has been shown to reduce serum testosterone and increase serum LH concentrations indicating an effect as an anti-androgen. Studies have yet to show if this effect translates to reduce hirsutism in practice.

inositol

The inositols are borderline substances that fall between food additives and medicinal products. Inositol was once thought to be part of the B groups of vitamins. D-chiro-inositol is a naturally occurring compound that makes insulin more effective – a similar effect to metformin. Myo-inositol is sold commercially as a nutritional supplement under the names *Inofolic* and *Pregnitude*.

There have been several studies that show that myo-inositol may have similar benefits to metformin. This treatment may work for women in whom metformin has little effect. Properly controlled research of high scientific quality is not available so it is hard to know what to advise about these compounds. If you are tempted to take this route then consider a defined therapeutic trial of a set duration such as three or six months to see if it makes a difference.

homoeopathy

Homoeopathy is a controversial area with the scientific community being critical of the concept of extremely dilute solutions being effective. Nevertheless, the long-standing reputation of this form of treatment makes it worth considering. The approach of homeopathy is often more holistic than that used by conventional doctors. The consultation is more wide-ranging which in itself may be of key importance in identifying stressors.

hypnosis

Hypnosis is popular but the effectiveness over the long-term is hard to judge. Intuitively this approach might be good for when there is a specific problem such as chocolate addiction or an unusual eating behaviour that prevents weight loss.

PCOS and eating disorders

Several studies have suggested a link between PCOS and eating disorders, particularly with bulimia. Other studies, notably those that included a well-characterised non-PCOS reference group, failed to show that bulimia was associated with PCOS. Nevertheless, eating patterns can have an effect on hormones and metabolism. Binge eating with intermittent fasts is thought to increase insulin concentrations and lower metabolic rate, which would both contribute to weight gain. Therefore, it seems likely that the link between the two conditions is that eating disorders may bring out symptoms of PCOS that would otherwise be slight. Treatment targeting an eating disorder therefore is likely to improve the symptoms of PCOS.

what is the best diet for women with PCOS?

There are many sources of information on diet and healthy eating for women with PCOS. In the end, you have to become your own expert to find the food combinations that you enjoy while at the same time feeling satisfied that you do not have to engage in constant mealtime battles between your hungry self and your healthy self. It is worth going over some of the fundamental principles of healthy eating. As mentioned above, one way of getting to know your food is by using an online diet diary to analyse the nutrient content – you may find that there are some surprises!

Little and often – the body processes food best if small amounts are taken at 3 to 4-hourly intervals. Beyond four hours, the body tends to shut down. It conserves energy instead of burning it. It takes only a small amount of calories to kick the system back into efficient burning. This is the reason why skipping breakfast is not a good idea. Try to spread food intake evenly throughout the day without any one meal being dominant. Make sure that 'little and often' does not add up to just 'more'!!

Keep it natural – anything that has been prepared for you or that comes packaged will tend to be high in sugar, fat and salt content because these components make food sell! Keeping a ready supply of natural food may take a little more time but can become a simple habit that improves weight control. For instance, having a ready supply of carrots, celery, cucumber and courgette available can help to fill in the gaps. Carbohydrate alternatives include rice cakes, oatcakes and crisp breads with toppings such as cottage cheese, light version of cream cheese or reduced-fat hummus.

Beware of apparently healthy food with hidden dangers – some of the biggest culprits in this group are the 'healthy' breakfasts. Muesli bars and granola cereals which can be very high in sugar and fat. It would be much better to take control of the ingredients to make your own alternatives.

Home preparation has the benefit of being able to cut sugar right back. Many recipes are just as good, if not better, with sugar content reduced by two thirds. Less obvious items in this category are the natural foods that are high in sugar including tropical fruit – melon, grapes and banana – dried fruit and fruit juices. While fine in moderation, these should be limited to one small portion per day. Other fruit such as apple and pear have a lower proportion of natural sugar.

Low glycaemic index foods – just having brown everything is not the whole story! Many people find that whole-wheat pasta is a step too far or that whole-meal bread can be indigestible. With regard to bread, have an experiment with gluten-free options that have improved greatly over the years. Try alternative types of grain such as spelt or buckwheat. Quinoa and flax have become popular super foods that help to make a substantial salad. Developing a taste for lentils and beans (not tinned baked beans steeped in sugar!) can be key to a satisfying low glycaemic index diet. As a reminder, it is the insoluble fibre in these pulses that keeps glucose in the gut longer so that it is released slowly. In addition, pulses are a good source of protein, folate and iron. If these are not already part of your diet, then it may be worth introducing them slowly, perhaps using them to pad out meat-based protein.

fasting diets

Fasting diets have become very popular as many people find this pattern easier than daily calorie restriction. This type of diet seems to be in conflict with the conventional advice to eat little and often and not to skip meals but it works for some people. Fasting diets involve eating normally for 5 days each week – say, 2000 kcal per day. Then for two 2 days – not consecutively – cut down to 500 kcal per day. There are many web sites offering recipes for the low calories days. Essentially these diet plans are low in fat and carbohydrate. It is amazing how much variety can be achieved using low fat proteins such as fish, chicken and egg with green vegetables and in soups.

The 5:2 diet has received a lot of attention for its medical benefits such as lowing blood sugar and blood pressure. With regard to PCOS, there are many enthusiasts reporting good results. In the end it is what works for you that matters so it is worth considering this option.

so, what can I eat?

As a starting point, the next table shows some meal-time suggestions. In order to find out what works well for you, be your own detective to find options that suit you. The basic format is protein with green leaf salad and green vegetables – these provide the filling cellulose component that can replace some of the carbohydrate.

Diet suggestions for women with PCOS

	Diet suggestion	Comment
Break-fast	Cereals – porridge, no added sugar muesli, Weetabix or shredded wheat	Inspect all cereal products carefully! Look for whole grain with no sugar
	Low fat yoghurt with fruit	
	Poached egg, grilled bacon and tomato with one slice of whole grain toast	If wheat is a problem then try other grains or rice cakes
Lunch	Mixed leaf salad with protein options – chicken, poached salmon, tinned tuna, boiled egg, lentils and beans, cottage cheese	Quinoa can be added to provide some slow release carbohydrate
	Lentils, beans, vegetables in the form of curry and rice, soup or chilli	Remembering to keep the rice portion small
	Salad-based wrap or sushi and salad	These are options that can be found in fast food outlets
Evening meal	Lean meat, chicken or fish with green vegetables such as green beans, cabbage, spring greens, kale, broccoli	Add a small portion of carbohydrate – wholegrain rice is probably the best – potatoes are not a good option. Try Puy lentils

Evening meal	Stir-fry using green vegetables and mushroom together with protein option. Use with rice noodles or try using finely cut or shredded courgette as an alternative.	Be careful with stir-fry sauces which can have added sugar – try making your own with soya sauce and only a small amount of honey
	Pasta sauce with added green vegetables.	Pasta need not be completely ruled out even in its white form. Instead of plates of pasta with a small amount of topping, try reversing this: a small amount of pasta with a more green vegetables
Extras	Low-calorie yoghurt with fresh fruit	
	Nuts and seeds	Although popular, keep an eye on the calorie content of nuts
	Water	Aim for a regular intake over the day
	Coffee and tea	Some people find that caffeine suppresses hunger. Others argue that these drinks are bad for metabolism. It is worth trying to stop for a while to test.

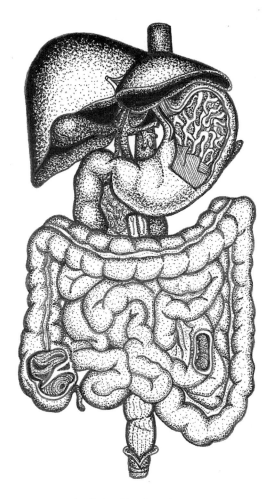

gastrointestinal system

This is the entire gastrointestinal system within the abdomen. Food enters at the top and leaves at the bottom! The large colon has been opened up on the lower left part very near the appendix that can just be seen. At the top is the liver on the left and just below that the stomach on the right, which has been opened to show the folded inner surface.

chapter 10
evolution and global aspects

If PCOS is related to infertility then why has it not died out over the years?

This question has been the focus of much thought. If women with PCOS have fewer children than others and if polycystic ovaries are genetically determined then there should be an evolutionary selection against the condition persisting in the population. PCOS should have been gradually eliminated from the world. For PCOS to be so common, there must be some survival benefit from having the genes that contribute to the condition.

evolutionary theory and PCOS

The first concept in this story is to imagine how PCOS might have behaved in an earlier era. In evolutionary terms, the last 50 years over which PCOS has come to scientific attention is only a small instant in time. In these 50 years our lifestyle has changed greatly. The epidemic of overweight has taken hold in many countries. Refined carbohydrate has only been commonplace for 100 years or so. Before the industrial revolution manual labour was the basis of most occupations. Even at home, physical work consumed most of the day. Therefore it may be that it is only recently that weight-related infertility has become a feature of PCOS. In an earlier age, when food supplies were low, many women who would have had PCOS in today's environment, might not have had any symptom or sign of the condition. In history therefore, there may have been no evolutionary pressure against PCOS. In the future generations, however, the impact of our modern lifestyle is likely to result in selection against PCOS were it not for the fact that modern treatments have ensured that the number of children from mothers with PCOS is normal.

The second concept to consider is why did PCOS evolve in the first place – what was the survival benefit? There are two ways to look at this. First, the genes that lead to the development of PCOS must also be related to genes that determine obesity and type 2 diabetes – the FTO gene for example. It might be important to have a group of individuals in a primitive community who store fuel efficiently as fat. It will be these people who survive a prolonged starvation. Others, without this genetic make-up may have become underweight and infertile from being too thin. For instance, periods often stop in women with low body weight.

This same principle explains why type 2 diabetes is becoming so common nowadays. If diabetes is bad for you then why has it not died out as a condition over time? Because it is only as the population grows fatter that evolutionary selection against diabetes becomes active. In the academic field of diabetes this is called the 'thrifty gene' concept. People who are thrifty with their energy supplies help a population survive starvation but become the group who acquire diabetes in times of plenty.

In summary, the overall priority of mankind is to have a diverse spectrum of individuals within the population, each with different genetic profiles in order to ensure the survival of the species. The greatest pressure over the evolution of mankind has been scarcity in the supply of food, so the ability to survive during times of starvation is a key requirement. Or to put it another way, populations who were not fortunate enough to have a scattering of PCO genes in their genetic pool have died out long ago. We have to thank women with PCOS for their forebears who allowed the species to survive!

expectation of modern times

One of the effects of having access to such a large amount of information on the Internet is that our expectations of what we should each be entitled to alters. The Internet has distorted our image of a perfect female appearance. The emphasis on celebrity as an ambition for young people has set unreasonable expectations. In a small community, a different appearance or behaviour may be easily absorbed. We are now comparing ourselves to an idealised vision of normal so we are likely to become more dissatisfied with our appearance. This is particularly true for the acceptability of body or facial hair. We appear to be passing through a time when complete absence of body hair is the ideal. This tendency may tempt women with PCOS to aim for greater clearance of excess hair growth with stronger drug treatments for a longer duration than previously. We may be entering unknown territory with this human experiment. Similarly, in order to keep up with this social trend, there is pressure to spend large amounts of money on hair removal treatments such as laser.

Achieving a sensible balance between expectation and achievable results is often an area that doctors do not cover well. Under pressure of time, many doctors will simply turn to the most effective prescription rather than consider the question of whether unreal expectations should be addressed. This leads one to think that more time spent on the psychology of making priorities in life may be more effective than conventional medical treatments.

PCOS around the world

Globally, PCOS has been found in every country and in all ethnic groups. In population studies using ovary ultrasound in women without obvious symptoms, it has been found that about 20% of women have more than 12 follicles in each ovary. That is, one fifth of all women qualify for the label of 'polycystic ovaries'. In some populations however, polycystic ovaries seems to be particularly common. In South Asia, screening with ultrasound has identified PCO in 50% of women. Interestingly this is also a population that has a high risk of diabetes and insulin resistance. This data mainly comes from studies in Sri Lanka but the same probably applies to women in India as well.

The South Asian population has an increased risk of developing type 2 diabetes. This means that, as a population, there will be a greater drive of insulin to the ovaries. Therefore, a greater proportion of women than expected would have polycystic ovary syndrome as opposed to polycystic ovaries with no symptoms. In addition, as the South Asian countries become more prosperous, there will be a big impact from weight gain leading to more symptoms of PCOS. There may be an evolutionary component here as well. In populations where food supplies have been limited, the metabolism has adjusted itself to being very economical with fuel – storing it efficiently as fat. As the same population begins to eat more, the bad effects from being overweight come on at a lower bodyweight than in a comparison group of Western women with PCOS.

From clinics in India, it is clear that women with relatively acceptable weight by western standards, say, a body mass index of 26 kg/m², show weight-related symptoms that a woman in the UK with a BMI of 35 kg/m² would be expected to have. This problem shows itself in fertility treatments. Women who are overweight can be resistant to simple fertility treatments such as clomifene citrate that becomes more effective as soon as weight loss begins. Therefore, for women in India with PCOS who are even slightly overweight, lifestyle measures will be more important than ever.

Most of the information from medical research that we have on treatments in PCOS comes from Europe and North America. Given that there are clear-cut metabolic differences between ethnic groups, it may be that the effectiveness of each treatment should be looked at separately in different regions of the world. For instance, in India, with a propensity to insulin resistance, it may be that metformin is more effective than in the West. This would also apply to other populations where insulin resistance is common including many indigenous populations such as aborigines, American Indians and Polynesian women with PCOS. This remains a completely unknown area that emphasises the fact that each region needs to develop local guidelines.

hair distribution around the world

One of the reference standards by which we quantify hair growth in women is the Ferriman-Gallwey score. This score was based on Caucasian women in the United Kingdom so it is not relevant for other populations. For instance, women from southern Mediterranean countries, from India and Sri Lanka tend to have more body hair compared to Caucasian women. However, the problem comes as to how society is judging you. For instance, an Indian woman in the UK may aspire to achieve a Caucasian hair distribution that might be quite difficult to achieve.

With regard to androgenic effects on the skin in different ethnic groups, Oriental women are much more prone to acne rather than hirsutism compared to other groups.

the obesity epidemic

Much of the Western world is in the grips of an epidemic of obesity that is now spreading globally. This of course will have a major impact on the management and presentation of PCOS. If we take it that 20% of all women have polycystic ovaries on ultrasound, then as the population becomes more obese so a greater proportion of this group will present with a symptom qualifying them for polycystic ovary <u>syndrome</u>. It has been suggested but not proven, that overweight itself may drive the development of polycystic ovaries especially if the weight comes on during childhood. If this is true then one might expect quite a marked rise in the prevalence of PCOS in the future.

In countries where obesity is very common, the whole agenda surrounding PCOS is based on weight control and the risk of diabetes. This is particularly true for information sources on the Internet where the USA predominates. For a lean woman with PCOS much of this information is not relevant. It is important to remember that PCOS also exists without obesity. In some clinics there has been such a focus on diabetes that insulin resistance appears to be found in almost every woman with PCOS depending on the criteria applied. As a consequence, Metformin is prescribed to nearly everyone even though it is often not effective. Also, some women have been told that they cannot have PCOS because they are not overweight!

In summary, as social trends change over time, so different features of PCOS become emphasised. Remember that PCOS is a personal thing and the best way forward has to be tailored on an individual basis.

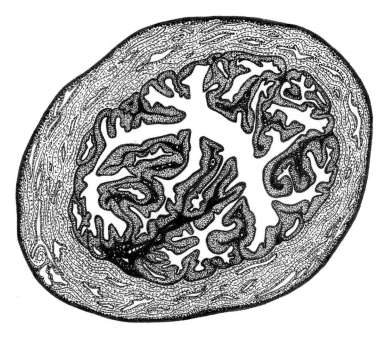

a fallopian tube

This is a cross-section of a fallopian tube which has a folded interior, on the surface of which are tiny hair-like cells that keep a flow of fluid that carries the egg from the ovary to the uterus. The wall of the fallopian tube is a ring of muscle and blood vessels. A fallopian tube is approximately 5 cm long and 2 mm wide. At the ovary end the tube opens out like a funnel with frond-like projections that are in contact with the ovary which make sure that the egg, once released, is firmly caught.

chapter 11

landmark papers and research

New information is coming in all the time. PCOS is one of the big enigmas in research, as we still do not know the fundamental cause of it. The risk of listing important papers is that they quickly go out of date and new ones will take their place. Nevertheless it is interesting to see how the concept of PCOS has changed over time – these changes are mainly driven by new technology.

This is a personal listing and not intended to be comprehensive. It is heavily influenced by my own research on insulin and the work of colleagues in the field. Also, I have dipped into the archives to find papers that marked a change in the understanding of PCOS.

I have chosen to list the papers by the year in which they were published. In this way, you can see how times have changed in relation to our understanding of PCOS. First, the name of the condition has changed over the years. Between 1935 and 1970 the literature favoured Stein-Leventhal Syndrome. After this polycystic ovarian <u>disease</u> was popular until ultrasound arrived on the scene in the 1980s and from then on PCOS became the most common term.

I have tried to seek out the first time that each formal system was described and also when each of the drug treatments were introduced. The intention is to provide a sense for the development of medicine and to show that nothing stands still – there will be more in the pipeline undoubtedly!

1935

Amenorrhea associated with bilateral polycystic ovaries.
Stein IF and Leventhal ML
American Journal of Obstetrics and Gynecolology, Volume: 29, Pages: 181–191.

I have chosen to begin the literature list with Stein and Leventhal whose names were given to the syndrome now called PCOS. Prior to this, there are occasional case reports particularly of bearded women but the clinical syndrome was brought together for the first time in this paper.

1949

Results of bilateral ovarian wedge resection in 47 cases of sterility; 20 year end results; 75 cases of bilateral polycystic ovaries.
Stein IF, Cohen MR and Elson R
American Journal of Obstetrics and Gynecolology, Volume: 58, Pages: 267–74.

Irving Stein continued his research with this major contribution describing the old technique of ovarian wedge resection that fell out of use some years later because of the surgical adhesions that would follow. Approximately one third of the ovary was removed in the early studies!

1957

Induction of human ovulation by individualized gonado–trophin therapy in two phases.
Igarashi M and Matsumoto S
American Journal of Obstetrics and Gynecolology, Volume: 73, Pages: 1294–8.

Using gonadotropins by injection to bring about ovulation began at about this time. With only minor adjustments over the years, this treatment is still used widely both for PCOS and for IVF.

1960

Urinary 17-ketosteroids in the syndrome of polycystic ovaries and hyperthecosis.
Lanthier A
Journal of Clinical Endocrinology and Metabolism, Volume: 20, Pages: 1587–600.

Before they could be measured in blood, androgens could be measured in urine as ketosteroids. This paper is one of the first that links high testosterone to polycystic ovaries. It is interesting that this is about 10 years before the focus turned to LH and then another 10 years after that before insulin came on the scene.

1961

Induction of ovulation with MRL/41. Preliminary report.
Greenblatt RB, Barfield WE, Jungck EC and Ray AW
JAMA, Vol: 178, Pgs: 101–4.

Before it was given the name clomifene, the first research on this fertility treatment used the name MRL-41. This paper marks the introduction of this treatment that remains the mainstay for infertility relating to PCOS over 50 years later!

1961

Clinical assessment of body hair growth in women.
Ferriman D and Gallwey JD
J Clin Endocrinol Metab, Volume: 21, Pages: 1440–7.

This is the famous scoring system to quantify hair growth in women – Ferriman and Gallwey score. It still remains one of the key research references even though it is rarely used in everyday practice.

1962

The polycystic ovary. I. Clinical and histologic features.
Goldzieher JW and Green JA
Journal of Clinical Endocrinology and Metabolism, Volume: 22, Pages: 325–38.

The reason why this paper is listed is because it brought together a large amount of clinical information and was the first to describe the appearance of the ovary from surgical specimens under the microscope.

1964

Gonadotropin therapy for the induction of ovulation.
Swyer GI
International Journal of Fertility, Volume: 9, Pages: 333–41.

I list this paper because Gerald Swyer preceded me at UCLH by a number of years. I never met him, but it is interesting that we must have overlapped in our clinical interest to a large degree. This is one of the first review papers describing the use of gonadotropins in infertility.

1969

The treatment of hirsutism with cyproterone acetate.
Hammerstein J and Cupceancu B
German Medical Monthly, Volume: 14, Pages: 599–602.

When I first attended clinic in the 1980s we used remarkably high doses of cyproterone acetate – up to 100 mg per day. The regimen of treatment was based on this paper written by the team who invented the concept of reverse sequential use of this antiandrogen. The reversed sequence referred to the fact that the drug was given in the first half of the menstrual cycle instead of the second half. Over time, we became more aware of the side-effects and the doses came down. Now I find that I rarely prescribe this compound.

1971

Serum gonadotropin levels and ancillary studies in Stein-Leventhal syndrome treated with clomiphene citrate.
Gambrell RD, Jr., Greenblatt RB and Mahesh VB,
Obstetrics and Gynecology, Volume: 38, Pages: 850–62.

It was only in the latter half of the 1960s that hormone levels for LH and FSH could be measured. This was one of the first papers that showed high LH as a characteristic feature of PCOS. 1971 was towards the end of the time that Stein-Leventhal syndrome was used as a diagnostic term.

1978

Spironolactone therapy for hirsutism in a hyperandrogenic woman.
Ober KP and Hennessy JF
Annals of Internal Medicine, Volume: 89, Pages: 643–4.

Spironolactone had been around for a number of years. Here is a paper that marks the introduction of spironolactone as an antiandrogen.

1983

Hyperandrogenism, insulin resistance, and acanthosis nigricans syndrome: a common endocrinopathy with distinct pathophysiologic features.

Barbieri RL and Ryan KJ,
American Journal of Obstetrics and Gynecolology, Volume: 147, Pages: 90–101.

This was one of the first papers that linked insulin resistance to androgen excess starting a whole new branch of research on the action of insulin on the ovary. In this paper, the subjects being overweight accounted for insulin resistance but it was the next paper in this year that sharpened the focus onto PCOS.

1983

Insulin resistance in non-obese patients with polycystic ovarian disease.
Chang RJ, Nakamura RM, Judd HL and Kaplan SA
Journal of Clinical Endocrinology and Metabolism, Volume: 57, Pages: 356–9.

Insulin resistance has always related to obesity but this was the first paper that showed raised insulin levels in women with PCOS who were of normal body weight. This was a turning point paper that started me on my research programme four years later.

1985

Multifollicular ovaries: clinical and endocrine features and response to pulsatile gonadotropin releasing hormone.
Adams J, Franks S, Polson DW, Mason HD, Abdulwahid N, Tucker M, Morris DV, Price J and Jacobs HS,
The Lancet, Volume: 2, Pages: 1375–9.

The introduction of high-resolution ultrasound in the 1980s made it possible to analyse the appearance of the ovary in more detail than was possible before. This paper is usually taken to be the one that first defined the polycystic ovary appearance using ultrasound even though it is the multifollicular that appears in the title. Multifollicular pattern is the one associated with low body weight and its distinction from polycystic ovaries remains a point of confusion still!

1989

Heterogeneity of the polycystic ovary syndrome: clinical, endocrine and ultrasound features in 556 patients.
Conway GS, Honour JW and Jacobs HS
Clinical Endocrinology, Volume: 30, Pages: 459–70.

At the time, this was one of the largest series of women with PCOS to be described. Along with subsequent papers, this work was initiated by my colleague and mentor Professor Howard Jacobs. Howard was the foremost clinical researcher in reproductive endocrinology in the UK and made an enormous contribution to the field particularly relating to PCOS.

1990

Effects of luteinizing hormone, insulin, insulin-like growth factor-I and insulin-like growth factor small binding protein 1 in the polycystic ovary syndrome.
Conway GS, Jacobs HS, Holly JM and Wass JA
Clinical Endocrinology, Volume: 33, Pages: 593–603.

This paper was my own effort at exploring the effect of insulin on the hormone balance in PCOS. It was this work that helped to formulate much of my thinking in clinic.

1992

Improvement in endocrine and ovarian function during dietary treatment of obese women with polycystic ovary syndrome.
Kiddy DS, Hamilton-Fairley D, Bush A, Short F, Anyaoku V, Reed MJ and Franks S

Clinical Endocrinology, Volume: 36, Pages: 105–11.

Even though weight loss is the most important form of treatment for women with PCOS there have been relatively few good papers demonstrating the benefit – this is one of the first and still referred to as a key paper. The comment is often made that the medical profession is more heavily influenced by drug trials than research into lifestyle!

1994

Clinical and hormonal effects of the 5 alpha-reductase inhibitor finasteride in idiopathic hirsutism.
Moghetti P, Castello R, Magnani CM, Tosi F, Negri C, Armanini D, Bellotti G and Muggeo M
Journal of Clinical Endocrinology abd Metabolism, Volume: 79, Pages: 1115–21.

This is the first of the good papers describing the use of finasteride for women with hirsutism who in current terminology would have had PCOS. It is interesting to look back on the timing of the use of new antiandrogens over the years.

1998

Polycystic ovary syndrome and insulin resistance: thrifty genes struggling with over-feeding and sedentary life style?
Holte J
Journal Endocrinological Investigation, Volume: 21, Pages: 589–601.

The effect of a modern lifestyle and evolutionary effect of thrifty genes was brought together in this key paper that introduced much of the thinking presented in chapter 10.

1998

Effects of metformin on spontaneous and clomiphene-induced ovulation in the polycystic ovary syndrome.
Nestler JE, Jakubowicz DJ, Evans WS and Pasquali R
New England Journal of Medicine, Volume: 338, Pages: 1876–80.

The use of Metformin in PCOS was first described in 1994 but it was this paper in 1998 that raised popular awareness. In retrospect, this was a very small study with a rather improbable success rate of 89% ovulation in those who took Metformin and 12% in those who did not. It took nearly 10 years before large-scale studies disproved a significant effect of metformin for fertility – see 2007.

1998

Mortality of women with polycystic ovary syndrome at long-term follow-up.
Pierpoint T, McKeigue PM, Isaacs AJ, Wild SH and Jacobs HS
Journal of Clinical Epidemiology, Volume: 51, Pages: 581–6.

It is extraordinarily difficult to gain a true picture of the possible effects of PCOS later in life. This landmark paper collected information from over 700 women with PCOS diagnosed between 1930 and 1979. The key finding was that there was no excess risk of heart disease despite the fact that the condition is associated with factors that might have said otherwise such as diabetes. There has been much debate about this conundrum over the years.

2004

Revised 2003 consensus on diagnostic criteria and long-term health risks related to polycystic ovary syndrome (PCOS).
Human Reproduction, Volume: 19, Pages: 41–7.

Although much debated, this consensus meeting provided a new definition of PCOS that has proved the test of time. A team of experts got together to define the ultrasound appearance and clinical features that would comprise the diagnosis of PCOS as outlined in chapter 2. This simple approach based on clinical features replaced previous criteria based on hormone measurements.

2003

Elevated serum level of anti-mullerian hormone in patients with polycystic ovary syndrome: relationship to the ovarian follicle excess and to the follicular arrest.
Pigny P, Merlen E, Robert Y, Cortet-Rudelli C, Decanter C, Jonard S and Dewailly D
Journal of Clinical Endocrinology and Metabolism, Volume: 88, Pages: 5957–62.

The hormone AMH had been around in research for some years and this paper was amongst the first showing elevated levels in PCOS. This group has also led the way in fine-tuning the science of counting follicles on ultrasound as their subsequent papers showed.

2007

Clomiphene, metformin, or both for infertility in the polycystic ovary syndrome.
Legro RS, Barnhart HX, Schlaff WD et. al.
New England Journal of Medicine, Volume: 356, Pages: 551–66.

This team raised the bar for fertility research by undertaking high quality large-scale studies using live birth rate as the outcome instead of the earlier and slightly misleading outcome of ovulation. After many years of research showing that metformin may be effective as a fertility treatment, this paper finally sealed the issue showing that Metformin was of no benefit if fertility was the most important issue.

2008

A systematic review of commonly used medical treatments for hirsutism in women.
Koulouri O and Conway GS
Clinical Endocrinology, Volume: 68, Pages: 800–5.

After realising that most of the information regarding treatment for hirsutism was based on very small poor quality studies, we wrote this paper in order to bring together everything we could find in the literature. The most important learning curve for me was that medical treatment for hirsutism became less effective as weight increased.

2009

Type 2 diabetes, cardiovascular disease, and the evolutionary paradox of the polycystic ovary syndrome: a fertility first hypothesis.
Corbett SJ, McMichael AJ and Prentice AM
American Journal of Human Biology, Volume: 21, Pages: 587–98.

For those readers interested in the section on evolution – this is the paper that explores this area the best. This is a variation on the "thrifty gene" hypothesis discussed in chapter 10. It makes for quite difficult reading but is rewarding in its explanation of how PCOS has persisted over evolution.

2009

The FTO gene modifies weight, fat mass and insulin sensitivity in women with polycystic ovary syndrome, where its role may be larger than in other phenotypes.
Kowalska I, Malecki MT, Straczkowski M et. al.
Diabetes and Metabolism, Volume: 35, Pages: 328–31.

It took 10 years from the discovery of this gene in 1999 to identify the link to PCOS. About one in seven Europeans carry two copies of this gene and on average they are 3 kg heavier that everyone else. This is the paper that links this genetic cause for obesity to PCOS.

2011

Genome-wide association study identifies susceptibility loci for polycystic ovary syndrome on chromosome 2p16.3, 2p21 and 9q33.3.
Chen ZJ, Zhao H, He L et. al.
Nature Genetics, Volume: 43, Pages: 55–9.

This paper is the first in a series of really large studies undertaking research to identify genes that contribute to the inheritance of PCOS. Over 4000 women with PCOS were included. A series of genes were identified in this paper and in those that followed. After many years of genetic research, this scale of endeavour may well begin to unravel the genetic cause of this syndrome.

2011

Risk of adverse pregnancy outcomes in women with polycystic ovary syndrome: population based cohort study.
RInternet N, Kieler H, Sahlin L, Ekman-Ordeberg G, Falconer H and Stephansson O
British Medical Journal, Volume: 343, Pages: d6309.

Using a medical register of over 3000 women with PCOS, this paper was the first to be large enough to show that polycystic ovary syndrome is a risk factor for diabetes in pregnancy even when bodyweight is taken into account. Before this paper, it was always a little unclear how much the association between gestational diabetes and PCOS could be accounted for by overweight.

2014

Letrozole versus clomiphene for infertility in the polycystic ovary syndrome
Legro RS, Brzyski RG, Diamond MP et. al.
New England Journal of Medicine, Volume: 371, Pages: 119–29.

This comparison of two fertility treatments is the first really good quality paper demonstrating a role for Letrozole. Letrozole has yet to come into routine practice in many centres simply because there is so much experience with clomiphene. This paper shows that Letrozole may be better than clomiphene for women who are overweight – BMI greater than 30 – but probably no better for women with a BMI less than 30.

acknowledgements

The first draft of this book was written in Kolhapur, India in a bungalow made available by my dear friend and colleague Dr Sachin Kulkani. Without that opportunity to spend two months in relative isolation but with wonderful catering, this project would never have lifted off the ground.

I can remember the early days of deciding whether to specialise in reproductive endocrinology, being unconvinced at first that there might be a career in it! I had the great good fortune of the mentorship of Professor Howard Jacobs. One of Howard's many skills is to encourage junior colleagues to develop by following their own enthusiasm. All of his junior fellows reflect on the stimulating Tuesday evening meetings when we debated the details of ultrasound and metabolism relating to PCOS. Much of the content of this book was handed down to me by HSJ.

There have been many who have helped in reading through various drafts of this book. There were my colleagues Melanie Davies, Anil Gudi, Tom King, Jennifer Ko, Vikram Talauliker and Ephia Yasmin. I was greatly assisted by patients who took this handbook on a trial run after the first draft and made many helpful suggestions.

On the production side, my wife Jane bravely took on the role of production manager! The long road of writing and revision was made possible entirely through Jane's encouragement and patient re-reading. Eleanor Scoones took on the detailed task of final proof reading and indexing. My assistant Maria Klasson has been invaluable in getting the final drafts in shape ready for publication.

Finally I would like to thank the many patients that I have met over the years who have shared their stories that collectively have turned into the contents of this book. Time spent in clinic listening to each person's experience has been a great privilege.

index